Contents

Foreword

Children still undergo unnecessary pain, distress, discomfort and suffering during the diagnosis and treatment of malignant disease. Although professional awareness of these issues is now much better, this book is in part a response to the fact that there is still some way to go. It is less often recognised that children treated for malignancy often suffer a heavy loss over and above their pain and distress: loss of belief in themselves as having control over their lives, loss of their sense of empowerment and loss of personal efficacy. Yet this too can be countered and managed, once it is acknowledged and understood. Children need not experience these losses, but if they do, the long-term consequences may be profound.

The strength of Christina Liossi's approach is its recognition of the inextricable link between the poor management of adverse experiences in childhood, and the subsequent ability of adults to cope adequately with adversity. Thus when children deal with the huge problem of malignancy and its treatment, the resilient ones may emerge unscathed, but others may be significantly harmed. So it is not enough merely to minimise pain and discomfort during the disease episode: we must look critically at how both pain and its management may help or harm children in the long term.

That it is not enough merely to judge procedural pain management on a unidimensional scale is illustrated through the story of the girl who preferred to be able to handle procedural discomfort through psychological techniques, rather than have a series of anaesthetics, because it gave her the control over the situation. As the passive recipient of anaesthesia, she was just that: a passive recipient. As someone who had learned a new technique to control her discomfort for herself, she had emerged from the experience with more than she had before. She illustrates that psychological management is not a bolt-on luxury for procedural pain management, it is central to an integrated and holistic approach to children's needs.

Reading this book you will be struck by the number of issues on which further research is needed, yet will see that much is known which can inform the practice of today and tomorrow. I have no doubt that you will reconsider the approaches and procedures in your own departments, and may be inspired to introduce new ones, underpinned by the broad range of evidence brought together here. You will be challenged by some pivotal ideas: I particularly liked the perspective of considering what a child actually knows, rather than starting from assumptions about what that child doesn't know. You will read the case histories and find that these stories give concrete expressions for some of the more abstract ideas.

But you may also be depressed by some details. So often in the case histories you will read about cases being referred for psychological evaluation, when things had clearly gone badly wrong for the child. Many of us will think, how come things were allowed to get that bad? This story is terrible, but we know it happens all too often – how can we get it right for every child? For there are never going to be enough psychologists to go round.

The challenge is, therefore, not one of finding more psychologists, nor one of educating professionals about when to refer. It is about embedding new ways of thinking, and new ways of working, in the multidisciplinary team. It is about the use of psychological techniques in parallel with pharmacology as a routine, not as an extra. It is about awareness of the child as an active participant, not a passive recipient. It is about arming key professionals – perhaps oncology nurses – with the right techniques so that they can evaluate the children themselves and help them directly. Precious resources such as a psychologist's time can then be used more efficiently in training and empowering others to prevent problems, rather than salvaging children who may already be psychologically harmed.

The gauntlet is thrown down. Christina Liossi shows us that we know what we need to do. We now have to find the means to do it.

Dr Martin Ward Platt MD, FRCPCH
Consultant Paediatrician and Senior Lecturer in Child Health
Royal Victoria Infirmary
Newcastle-upon-Tyne
October 2001

Foreword

In the last two decades, unprecedented scientific and clinical attention has focused on the special pain problems of children. Extensive research has created better insights into how children perceive pain and how clinicians can alleviate their suffering. However, under-treated pain continues to be a major problem for many infants, children and adolescents. A large gap still exists between what we know about controlling children's pain and how we practise clinically, and the control of post-operative pain, cancer pain, painful sickling crises, and chronic pain remains problematic for children in many centers.

The control of cancer pain, both pain from metastatic disease and pain from necessary cancer treatments, remains a serious health concern. Optimal pain control for children with cancer begins with the recognition that children's pain is not simply and directly related to the extent of their physical injuries or the severity of their disease. Many factors can modify the neural signals for pain and increase a child's pain and distress. As for adults, children's pain perception depends upon complex neural interactions, where impulses generated by tissue damage are modified both by ascending systems activated by innocuous stimuli and by descending pain-suppressing systems activated by various situational and psychological factors.

Our increasing appreciation of the plasticity and complexity of children's pain has profound implications for pain management. Since a child's pain is not wholly determined by the level of tissue damage, we cannot completely control pain by gearing our interventions solely to the putative source of tissue damage. Instead, we must also identify the situational and psychological factors that can cause or exacerbate a child's pain and target our interventions accordingly. Controlling children's pain requires a dual emphasis on administering appropriate analgesics or anaesthetics, and on selectively modifying the factors that exacerbate their pain. Our treatment emphasis thus should shift from an exclusive disease- or procedure-centered focus to a more child-centered focus. The challenge for the future is to integrate this child-centered approach more efficiently into clinical practice.

Christina Liossi is helping us to meet this challenge. This comprehensive text provides a clear framework for understanding how children perceive pain, how we can assess their pain, and how we can better select drug and non-drug therapies to alleviate pain caused by medical procedures. Information on the factors unique to cancer pain, as well as those common to many types of acute procedure-related pain, enables healthcare providers to better understand their profound role in mediating a child's pain and distress. Emphasis in clinical care has often been placed more on helping children to cope with or endure painful treatments than on alleviating the pain evoked by treatments. Perhaps healthcare providers have accepted too thoroughly the assumption that pain is inevitable during noxious procedures.

However, as described throughout this text, we have effective drug and non-drug therapies for procedure-related pain, child-centered programmes, and innovative ideas for implementing treatment guidelines in clinical practice. Thus, healthcare providers can develop a diverse repertoire of practical non-drug methods to complement 'state of the art' drug management. They can adopt evidence-based guidelines for selecting the most appropriate drugs to control pain caused by the varied procedures children receive during their cancer treatment. Moreover, healthcare providers can integrate many versatile, inexpensive, and effective pain-reducing methods into routine clinical practice so as to target all the causative and contributing factors for children's pain. In this manner, we can truly provide optimal pain control to the children entrusted to our care.

Professor Patricia A McGrath
Professor of Pediatrics
Faculty of Medicine
University of Western Ontario
October 2001

Preface

Pain in general and procedure-related pain in particular are important considerations in the care of children with cancer. Although there have been improvements in pain treatment over the last few decades, there are numerous studies documenting the fact that unrelieved procedure-related pain is still prevalent in paediatric oncology. Indeed, procedure-related pain management continues to be an extremely challenging problem for the young sufferers, their families and healthcare professionals alike. Research has demonstrated that children with cancer and their parents regard invasive procedures as one of the most difficult aspects of having cancer, and their distress and recollections of these traumatic events persist years after the completion of anti-cancer treatment.

This book provides a concise overview of essential theory and techniques for the assessment and management of procedure-related pain in children and adolescents with cancer, clearly illustrated with case histories. The book provides the theoretical knowledge required to understand the specific nature and assessment strategies of procedure-related cancer pain, and it describes and discusses in depth both pharmacological and psychological methods of pain relief, together with the difficulties that may be encountered in their implementation. Clinical and research material gathered over the last 10 years from my clinical work in paediatric oncology and palliative care can be found throughout the book.

Two themes underlie this book. The first is that psychological and pharmacological interventions should be better combined and form a comprehensive, integrated approach to the clinical management of paediatric procedure-related cancer pain. My goals include raising awareness and educating where necessary that psychological techniques as implemented by healthcare professionals are a powerful adjunct to pharmacological intervention, and encouraging their more frequent and consistent use in paediatric cancer settings.

The second theme is that there should be closer integration between research work and clinical practice. It is my intention that this book will bridge the gap between research and clinical practice and will have direct application to the clinical environment. The aim was to write a book for practitioners who desire information about the most effective, empirically documented methods of procedure-related pain assessment and management that can be applied in the clinical area. Moreover, the details presented should inform clinical investigators about a number of areas in which clinical insights have revealed important issues that are in need of empirical testing and support.

In Chapter 1, the physiology and psychology of procedure-related cancer pain are reviewed, and a cognitive–behavioural framework for understanding pain is provided. In Chapter 2, the most psychometrically sound, practical and widely used pain assessment and measurement methods are described and the reader is given simple suggestions with regard to their role and use in a busy oncology setting. Chapter 3 focuses on the pharmacological management of procedure-related pain, and analgesic interventions such as local anaesthesia, general anaesthesia and conscious sedation are described and guidelines for their safe and effective implementation in the paediatric oncology setting are provided. Chapters 4 and 5 provide a concise review of the most effective and widely used psychological interventions for the management of procedure-related cancer pain in clinical practice. Interventions such as preparation, distraction, cognitive therapy and hypnosis are described in considerable detail, with the aim of familiarising the professional who would like to incorporate them into their clinical practice. The final chapter is devoted to the integration of the pharmacological and psychological analgesic interventions, providing realistic and practical suggestions and protocols for achieving this in the clinical setting.

Although the comprehensive and intensive approach described in this book was developed, researched and applied primarily for the complex needs of the child with cancer, variations of the approaches can be applied to those young patients with other disorders who have to undergo repeated painful procedures, such as children with kidney failure undergoing dialysis, children with diabetes, and those who as part of a treatment for any condition have to undergo painful or stressful medical procedures.

I am grateful to the many people who kindly supported and encouraged me, provided technical assistance, critically discussed ideas or reviewed the manuscript. In particular, I wish to thank Dr Richard Hain, Professor Popi Hatira, Dr Mary Haslum, Mr Peter Durnin, Dr Roula Liossi and Dr Robert Twycross. My young patients and their parents have throughout the years provided me with insights into their private world of pain and cancer, have participated in my research studies and have given me some of their drawings to include in this book. I offer them my respect and heartfelt affection. Finally, I would like to acknowledge the help and support I have received from the staff of Radcliffe Medical Press, and I would like to thank Miss Popi Chalkidou for her skilful secretarial assistance.

Christina Liossi
October 2001

About the authors

Christina Liossi BA, MPhil, CPsychol
Lecturer in Health Psychology
University of Wales, Swansea

Richard Hain MBBS, MSc, MD, MRCP, FRCPCH, Dip Pall Med
Honorary Consultant in Paediatric Oncology
Senior Lecturer in Paediatric Palliative Care
University of Wales College of Medicine, Cardiff

1

The nature of paediatric procedure-related cancer pain

Christina Liossi

Introduction

The last few years have represented an incredibly exciting period for pain research in general and paediatric pain research in particular. Major advances have occurred in the understanding of pain, and in the development and refinement of pain measures, as well as in the use of effective pain control methods. An adequate review of each of these developments is beyond the scope of this book. Instead, this and subsequent chapters will provide a brief overview of the state of the art with regard to pain in children,[1.1] with the emphasis on procedure-related cancer pain. In this chapter the physiological and the cognitive models of pain will be described in detail and the implications of this conceptualisation of pain for pain assessment and management will be explored.

Paediatric cancers

Childhood cancers are comparatively rare, affecting 1 in 600 children before the age of 15 years. However, with the decline in fatal childhood infections, the proportion of deaths due to cancer has risen. Cancer is now the second commonest cause of death in children between the ages of 1 and 14 years, after trauma. Each year in the UK there are around

1.1   Throughout the book the generic term 'children' is used to denote child and adolescent groups.

1300 new childhood cancer patients – that is, an annual incidence rate[1.2] of 1 per 10 000 children. In the USA, about 6550 new cases of cancer are diagnosed annually in children under the age of 15 years, and about 2175 deaths occur. Childhood cancer occurs slightly more commonly in boys than in girls (M : F ratio 1.3 : 1). The commonest childhood cancers are the leukaemias, which represent a third of all cancers.[1]

The outlook for children with cancer has improved radically since the widespread introduction of combination chemotherapy in the late 1960s and early 1970s. Before that time very few cancers could be treated effectively,[2] but now at least half are probably cured, and for many types the survival rates are much higher (up to 75%). For example, the 5-year survival rate for acute lymphoblastic leukaemia, the commonest childhood cancer, has increased sevenfold, from 9% in 1962–70 to 70% for children treated in the period 1983–85.[3]

Psychosocial issues of paediatric cancer

As survival rates of paediatric cancer have increased,[4] awareness of the psychological needs of the patient and their family has improved. The child's adaptation during disease and treatment and his or her quality of life as a long-term survivor are of paramount concern. For the child with cancer, successful outcome in all psychosocial domains depends on early assessment, prevention and intervention. Psychosocial issues associated with the diagnosis of cancer frequently include fears of death and separation. Treatment of cancer may also cause negative side-effects such as pain, nausea and vomiting, and loss of hair. These side-effects, as well as fears and anxieties, may impact negatively on treatment compliance, which in turn affects disease outcome.[5] Furthermore, if treatment is offered at a regional hospital some distance from the child's home, the child may be obliged to miss school and to be separated from family and friends. Box 1.1 summarises some of the common psychological problems that are experienced by children with cancer.

The diagnosis and treatment of cancer have an equally significant impact on the child's family. Siblings of the paediatric cancer patient may experience guilt, isolation and envy of the sick child's special attention and privileges. Parents experience a wide range of feelings, including anger, sadness and guilt, as well as fears about their child's illness, treatment, side-effects or potential death.[6] The stress of a child's cancer is

---

1.2   The cancer incidence rate is the number of new cases in a given time interval divided by the population at risk.

Box 1.1: Sources of psychological distress in children with cancer

Disease	Rapidly progressive, shortened life expectancy, unrelieved pain, uncontrolled symptoms, disfigurement, disabilities, physical dependence, long illness leading to psychological exhaustion
Treatment	Diagnostic delays, and multiple, stressful failed treatments
Patient	Fear of pain, dying, disfigurement, impaired sexuality, loss (or fear of loss) of control, independence and dignity, feelings of helplessness, hopelessness, insight regarding (or fear of) poor prognosis, loss of self-esteem, loss (or fear of loss) of school, social position or family role, feelings of isolation (actual or perceived)
Social	Pre-existing family problems, lack of peer interaction and support
Treatment team	Poor communication, unhelpfulness, lack of interest, lack of information, lack of continuity of care, exclusion of family

---

likely to exacerbate any problems that are already present in a marriage or family, such as poor communication, poor problem solving, or financial difficulties. The majority of paediatric oncology centres, recognising the problems inherent in the situation, are currently offering psychosocial services both to their patients and to the families concerned.

Epidemiology of paediatric cancer pain

Pain is a commonly encountered problem in the care of children and adults with cancer. Numerous studies have documented a high incidence of pain in adults with cancer.[7] However, these data cannot always be generalised to children, since adults differ with regard to factors such as growth, development and types of malignant disease. Chronic, debilitating pain is not encountered as often in children with cancer as in adults, because of the nature of the malignancy. Therefore the categories developed for the different types of adult cancer pain do not accurately characterise children's cancer pain. Procedure-related pain in children demands a category of its own. It is a potent source of discomfort and anxiety in the paediatric patient – much more so than in the adult. A useful classification for children has been proposed by Ljungman *et al.*,[8] who suggest that cancer pain can be reduced to one or more of four basic aetiologies as follows:

- cancer related (e.g. pain due to infiltration of the tumor in various organs or tissues)
- treatment related (e.g. pain as a side-effect of chemotherapy and radiation – for example, mucositis, radiation dermatitis, drug-induced peripheral neuropathy, prolonged post-lumbar puncture headache)
- procedure related (e.g. pain due to finger-prick, venepuncture, lumbar puncture, bone-marrow aspiration and trephine, or post-operative pain)
- pain of other aetiology (e.g. growth pains, trauma).

Few studies have carefully addressed the incidence of pain in children with cancer. Miser[9] reported that 60–70% of adults with cancer experience pain that is directly related to their cancers, while in children direct pain occurs in only about 25% of cases. Painful episodes are more likely to be due to therapy and procedures (50% of cases). A significant amount of pain (25% of cases) is completely unrelated to the cancer itself. Most children with cancer experience pain which, like the progression of cancer in children, differs from that in adults. After diagnosis, the common childhood malignancies generally respond rapidly to treatment, and disease-related pain often remits. If cancer recurs and is resistant to treatment, the disease progresses rapidly, resulting in early death after a relatively short palliative phase.

Procedure-related pain in children with cancer

Even if cancer is not painful in its own right, young patients with cancer undergo numerous painful procedures as part of diagnosis, therapy and supportive care, including venepuncture (VP), lumbar puncture (LP), bone-marrow aspiration (BMA) and trephine.[1,3] A typical Children's Cancer Group protocol for standard-risk acute lymphoblastic leukaemia requires more than 20 lumbar punctures or bone-marrow aspirations throughout the course of treatment.[10] Epidemiological studies of the pain associated with chronic disease suggest that, for many children, the pain associated with procedures is the most distressing part of their disease,[11,12] and frequent repetition of procedures does not desensitise them to the distress.[13,14] In fact, during the past decade, a growing body of scientific evidence has suggested that the diagnosis of such a threatening condition as cancer, followed by the exhausting procedures

1.3   The relevant painful and non-painful procedures are described in detail in Chapter 3.

imposed by highly technical investigations and treatments, are stressors which are potentially responsible for significant psychological distress, anxiety and depression, which negatively affect personal well-being and social functioning, and which may represent an obstacle to treatment compliance.[15] It is therefore essential for all children with cancer that intervention for suffering includes concern about and management of the pain and distress associated with procedures. Furthermore, routinely teaching paediatric oncology patients the skills necessary to cope with painful procedures and cancer treatment in general before problems develop can decrease their anxiety and distress considerably, increase their self-esteem and enhance their quality of life.

One would think that the obvious and persistent distress that procedures generate in children would have elicited from the medical, psychological and nursing communities various pharmacological and psychological strategies aimed at eradicating this problem. This has not historically been the case. It is clear from US studies conducted in the mid-1980s[16,17] that most cancer centres for children did not use premedication for bone-marrow aspirations or biopsies. In a survey performed in 1987,[16] only 30% of centres used routine premedication for children undergoing bone-marrow aspirations or biopsies. When medication was used, it was most frequently the Demerol/Phenergan/Thorazine (DPT) cocktail – a concoction developed in the 1950s for cardiac catheterisations, which requires an intramuscular injection, has a relatively high incidence of associated side-effects,[18,19] and causes prolonged sedation. The second most widely used agent was chloral hydrate – a hypnotic agent with no analgesic properties. When Homan and colleagues[20] surveyed members of the Pediatric Oncology Group in 1991, they found that 75% of children received premedication prior to their bone-marrow aspirations, and DPT was still the most commonly used agent for sedation, with midazolam – a short-acting benzodiazepine that offers no analgesia but has strong amnestic properties – as the second commonest choice. Although there has clearly been an improvement, 25% of children did not receive premedication, and many received an inappropriate or inadequate drug regimen. It appears that some aspects of paediatric pain management have improved considerably, but the management of pain during diagnostic and treatment procedures continues to be variable and often inadequate.[21]

Paediatric cancer patients frequently protest about venepunctures, bone-marrow aspirations, lumbar punctures and even painless procedures such as CT scans. The anxiety and distress generated in anticipation of these procedures are sometimes so severe that children (and often also their parents) exhibit symptoms such as nausea, vomiting, insomnia, nightmares and skin rashes prior to the procedure. The degree of behavioural distress and lack of co-operation observed during a procedure ranges from nuisance to major management problems. Behaviours such as crying, screaming and physical resistance create additional stress for parents, clinicians and any other children present. Young children often exhibit their distress during procedures to such an extent that physical restraint is necessary and it is very difficult for the medical staff to perform the procedures. Experiencing a procedure that is stressful often leads to feelings of anxiety and fear, and a vicious cycle of fear, anxiety and distress/pain may then develop. Zeltzer and LeBaron,[22] as the initial part of a study looking at behavioural interventions for procedure-related pain, asked 33 children between the ages of 6 and 17 years to rate on a visual analogue scale (VAS) from 1 to 5 (where 1 = no pain and 5 = the worst pain imaginable) the amount of pain and anxiety associated with lumbar punctures and bone-marrow aspirations. Children's rating for pain during bone-marrow procedures was 4.51, and that during lumbar punctures was 3.7. They rated anxiety during bone-marrow aspirations as 4.2 and during lumbar punctures as 3.75. It is clear that these common procedures cause an enormous amount of distress in children, and for many of them they represent the worst part of having cancer.

Katz and colleagues,[23] and Jay and colleagues[24] also studied children's responses to painful diagnostic procedures. They found that distress was inversely related to age – that is, the younger the child, the greater the distress demonstrated during the procedure. Jay *et al.*[24] found that levels of distress were five times higher in young children than in older children, with a dramatic decrease in distress at approximately 6 to 7 years of age, at which time children could cognitively understand the need for these procedures, as well as the notion that short-term discomfort might have a long-term benefit. However, even older children had significant concerns about these procedures.

Inadequately treated procedure pain increases anxiety about subsequent clinical encounters, which may in turn increase pain. Following a placebo-controlled randomised clinical trial to assess the efficacy of oral transmucosal fentanyl for children undergoing bone-marrow aspiration or biopsies,[25] the entire group (both the initial placebo group and the active group) received transmucosal fentanyl for subsequent procedures. It was found that the young children who had an initial negative experience (the placebo group) reported more pain during their subsequent procedures than the group who had experienced less pain initially (the active drug group).[26] Despite continued preparation and active drug, it was impossible to eradicate the anxiety and sense of dread that the children in the placebo group brought to the next procedure, which increased their perception of pain. However, children over 8 years of age did not show a similar pattern.

This research finding is consistent with clinical experience and developmental theory. Young children who have had a negative experience resulting from inadequate analgesia might anticipate that their next experience will be similarly negative. Given their developmental level and cognitive capabilities, they are less likely to benefit from preparation. In comparison, older children who operate at a different cognitive level can understand that the medication which they receive the next time may be more effective, and that recurrent painful experiences are not inevitable.[26] The data therefore suggest that when analgesics are used, it is critically important that they should be effective the first time, especially for younger children. This argues against the traditional strategy of selecting a lower dose and titrating upward.

It is the obligation of health professionals caring for children who require multiple procedures to manage the pain associated with those procedures aggressively from the beginning. During subsequent procedures, the treatment plan can be individualised for each child depending on the child's personality, specific disease, family and social variables, as well as other characteristics. However, it is crucial that appropriate and adequate analgesia is given from the outset, so that the parents and child who are already struggling with the enormous change that a cancer diagnosis brings in their lives do not have to bear the additional burden of preventable pain.

Today, as this book amply demonstrates, effective, well-documented, combined, comprehensive, psychological and pharmacological approaches are available. Adequate doses of appropriate drugs that are effective in suppressing the experience of pain are used together with psychological measures that are effective in raising the threshold for the experience of pain. The basis for this comprehensive multidisciplinary approach is a thorough assessment of the whole child and his or her family.

Pain defined

The most widely accepted definition of pain today is that developed by the International Association for the Study of Pain.[27] It states that 'pain is an unpleasant sensory and emotional experience associated with actual or potential tissue damage, or described in terms of such damage. Pain is always subjective.' This definition encompasses both

Box 1.2:   The subjective nature of pain[28]
Pain is whatever the experiencing person says it is, existing whenever he says it does.

sensory (i.e. nociception) and emotional (i.e. suffering) factors. It also draws on both 'actual' and 'potential' events. The definition blurs potentially observable indications of damage with unobserved descriptions when it states 'described in terms of such damage'. The idea that 'pain is always subjective' is very important, and highlights the fact that pain is a somatopsychic experience (see Box 1.2).

This definition also highlights the fact that pain is an unpleasant experience with both 'sensory' and 'emotional' aspects. The sensory aspect of pain refers to the stimulation and activation of specialised sensory receptors in the nervous system by noxious stimuli.[29-31] The activation of these receptors creates nociceptive sensory input, and this in turn is transformed neurochemically into nerve signals. Specific neural pathways in the spinal cord transmit these signals to the brain, where they are interpreted.[29-32] Psychological factors affect the way in which a person interprets or perceives these signals of noxious stimulation and, conversely, perceptions of the noxious stimuli determine that person's psychological reactions to the physical sensations. This conceptualisation emphasises that pain is more a perception than a sensation, and that it is mediated by sensory, physiological, cognitive, emotional, behavioural and contextual factors. Because the perception of pain is an individual experience, no two people can feel pain in exactly the same way. Similarly, a person's perception of pain at different points in time is likely to vary as a result of psychological and contextual variables.

Acute pain may be defined as 'pain of recent onset and probable limited duration'.[31,33,34] Typically, it has an identifiable temporal and causal relationship with a physical injury or disease process (e.g. pain associated with a broken arm, post-surgical pain). Thus acute pain begins with a physical insult to some structures or tissues of the body, and is time limited to hours, days or weeks. Its intensity is usually greatest at the time of onset. As healing or tissue repair takes place, there is usually a corresponding gradual reduction in nociception and acute pain sensation. By definition, acute pain eventually remits, either spontaneously or with some form of treatment that addresses the associated injury or disease. Acute pain may be accompanied by anxiety and clinical signs of sympathetic overactivity such as tachycardia, tachypnoea, hypertension, sweating, papillary dilatation and pallor. Chronic pain according to Bonica[35] persists one month beyond the usual course of an acute disease or a reasonable time for an injury to heal, or is associated with a chronic pathological process which causes continuous pain or pain which recurs at intervals for months or years. Chronic pain patients appear depressed and withdrawn and, as there are usually no signs of sympathetic over-activity, sometimes they appear to be free of pain.[1.4]

Acute pain serves to notify a person of present or potential physical harm (e.g. a fractured ankle, a burned finger, physical exhaustion from overactivity). Because acute pain offers biologically protective information about the need to remove oneself from harm and to address the cause of the discomfort, it is a primary symptom that motivates people to act.[34] However, when pain persists long after it has served its primary signalling function, it can impair the quality of life.

Psychological and contextual variables mediate a person's response to acute pain. Many factors affect people's psychological responses, including the understood cause of the pain, the circumstances of its onset, its understood medical prognosis and memories of previous pain experiences.[36] Acute (recent-onset) and subacute (relatively recent-onset) pain associated with strong negative emotions such as fear, grief or anger can persist long after a precipitating physical injury has been treated.[37] Furthermore, pain experienced in a context (e.g. hospital) that triggers strong negative emotions, feelings of lack of control or conflictual feelings (e.g. guilt, anger, secondary gains) can impair a person's recovery from pain.[38] With emotional lives that are disrupted severely by cancer and in an environment that is far from child friendly in the majority of cases, many children understandably become anxious, angry and depressed in response to even the simplest procedures, which may not in fact be painful (e.g. a CT scan).

Researchers who adopt a neurophysiological and neuroanatomical approach have identified mechanisms that detect and transmit information about noxious stimuli to the dorsal horn of the spinal cord, and mechanisms there that receive, interpret and transmit messages to the brain.[35] However, others have shown that no fixed relationship exists between excitation of particular afferent categories and behavioural outcomes.[39] It has also been shown that the input and output of individual dorsal horn cells are not related. The attenuated relationship between peripheral stimulation and spinal sensory processing is in part a product of the plasticity of the nervous system. Thus neurophysiologically and neuroanatomically based evidence indicates that pain behaviours or responses have a variable relationship to nociceptive stimulation. For

---

1.4   Some useful pain-related terms include the following: *sensation threshold*, the least stimulus at which a person perceives a sensation; *pain threshold*, the least experience of pain which a subject can recognise; *pain tolerance*, the greatest level of pain which a subject is prepared to tolerate.

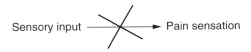

Figure 1.1:   The sensory input–pain sensation relationship.

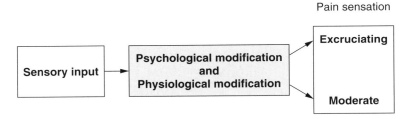

Figure 1.2:   The sensory input–pain sensation relationship.

any given noxious stimulus, the pain experienced may vary widely as a result of psychological variables. Therefore Figure 1.1 is incorrect, whereas Figure 1.2 depicts reality.

Pain physiology

Pain is a complex sensory and cognitive experience which is interpreted at the level of the cerebral cortex, and the signal that is interpreted as pain can arise at any point in the pain pathway (*see* Figure 1.3). The route by which a noxious stimulus initiates the perception of pain can be considered anatomically at a number of levels:[1.5]

- nociceptors
- primary afferent conduction
- dorsal horn
- ascending tracts
- descending modulation of pain
- neurotransmitters
- neural plasticity.

Nociceptors

Noxious stimuli activate specific pain receptors (nociceptors) in the tissues, which transform pain information into an electrical signal which

1.5   Here only somatic pain will be considered. Readers interested in visceral and sympathetically maintained pain are referred to Doyle *et al.*[40] and Twycross.[41]

PERCEPTION

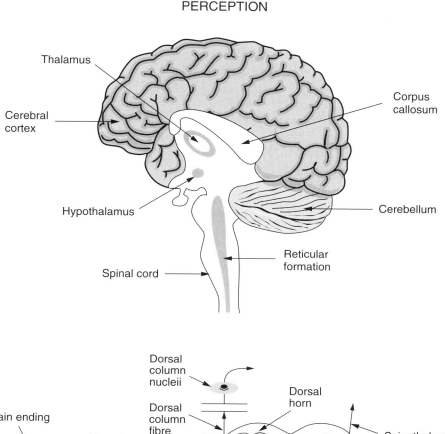

Figure 1.3: The pain pathway.

is conducted centrally. Like other cutaneous and subcutaneous receptors, nociceptors transduce a variety of stimuli into receptor potentials, which in turn trigger afferent action potentials. Nociceptors are normally inactive, but are excited by mechanical, thermal and chemical stimuli. Unless sensitised they respond only to noxious, or potentially noxious, stimuli. Moreover, nociceptors, like other somatic sensory receptors, arise from cell bodies in dorsal root ganglia (or in the trigeminal ganglion) that send one axonal process to the periphery and the other into the spinal cord or brainstem. Because peripheral nociceptive axons terminate in unspecialised 'free endings', it is conventional to categorise nociceptors according to the properties of the axons associated with them.

There are two types of free nerve endings of unmyelinated and finely myelinated neurones. One group responds to mechanical deformation, and these are known as high-threshold mechanoreceptors. The others respond to a variety of noxious inputs and are known as polymodal nociceptors. A number of chemicals are involved in the stimulation and sensitisation of polymodal receptors, including hydrogen ions, bradykinin, histamine, prostaglandins, leucotrienes, 5HT and cytokines. The receptors (and the fibres of which they are the free nerve endings) are the Aδ (alpha-delta; finely myelinated) and the C (unmyelinated) primary afferent fibres. The Aδ fibres, which conduct at about 20 m/s, are spread in the body surface, muscles and joints and give rise to rapid, pricking, well-localised pain. C fibres, which conduct at velocities generally less than 2 m/s, can be found in most tissues and are associated with slow, diffuse, dull, aching pain. Thus, even though the conduction of all nociceptive information is relatively slow, there are fast and slow pain pathways. The 'first' or 'fast' sharp pain which one experiences when pinpricking a finger is mediated by Aδ fibres. The 'second' or 'slow' diffuse, throbbing, possibly burning pain which follows seconds later and lasts longer is mediated by C fibres. A common property of both Aδ and C fibres is sensitisation when exposed to repeated noxious stimuli. The receptive fields of all pain-sensitive neurones are relatively large, particularly at the level of the thalamus and cortex, presumably because the detection of pain is more important than its precise localisation.

Primary afferent conduction

Like the other sensory neurones in dorsal root ganglia, the central terminations of Aδ and C fibres enter the spinal cord via the dorsal roots. The majority enter the dorsal horn in the ventrolateral bundle of the dorsal root – lateral to the larger-diameter myelinated Aβ fibres (alpha-beta). Approximately 30% of the central processes of unmyelinated fibres enter the spinal cord through the ventral root, and they also terminate in the dorsal horn of the cord. When these centrally projecting axons reach the dorsal horn, they branch into ascending and descending collaterals, forming the dorsolateral tract of Lissauer (named after the

German neurologist who first described this pathway in the late nineteenth century). Axons in Lissauer's tract run up and down for one or two spinal cord segments before they penetrate the grey matter of the dorsal horn.[42]

Dorsal horn

The dorsal horns of the spinal cord are divided into (Rexed) laminae on the basis of their histological appearance (these laminae are description divisions of the spinal grey matter in cross section, named after the neuroanatomist who described these details in the 1950s). Although the laminae have discrete functions related to pain processing, there are numerous connections between them. Lamina II, the substantia gelatinosa, extends from the trigeminal nucleus in the medulla to the filum terminale. C fibres terminate in lamina II. They synapse predominantly with small second-order neurones, most of which synapse again within the segment of entry or within the two adjacent segments. Because of their short length they are sometimes called 'interneurones'. $A\delta$ fibres terminate in laminae I and V. $A\beta$ fibres (low-threshold cutaneous and deep-muscle mechanoreceptors), which respond to innocuous stimuli such as vibration and light touch, enter the cord medial to the dorsal horn and pass without synapse to the dorsal columns. However, they give off collateral branches to the dorsal horn which terminate in several laminae, particularly III–V and deeper. They also synapse directly with terminals of unmyelinated C fibres in lamina II. There they can release gamma-aminobutyric acid (GABA), which inhibits C-fibre transmission. The laminae II and V that receive afferent input from both large- and small-diameter fibres are important sites for pain modulation and localisation. The two subgroups subserve different functions. The superficial second-order neurones are involved in pain localisation, whereas the deeper ones are involved with coding pain intensity. However, both cross the spinal cord and ascend in the contralateral anterolateral tract to the brainstem, and in some cases to the thalamus. From lamina III and deeper, information is summated from direct input from the periphery and from more dorsal laminae.

The extent to which painful peripheral stimuli are conducted centrally and perceived as pain depends on the degree to which two major modulating mechanisms at the level of the dorsal horn 'close the gate' to onward transmission. In the first of these, activity in large myelinated afferent ($A\beta$) fibres is via inhibitory circuits in the superficial laminae of the dorsal horn to suppress transmission in small unmyelinated (C-fibre) afferents. In the second mechanism, inhibitory control from higher centres is tonically active.[42] The dorsal horn, particularly the substantia gelatinosa, contains several neurotransmitters, including substance P, glycine, GABA and enkephalins. The substantia gelatinosa is one of the densest neuronal areas in the central nervous system (CNS), and is crucial for the reception and modulation of nociceptive messages delivered by peripheral fibres.

Ascending tracts

From the dorsal horn, nociceptor neurones ascend in the contralateral spinothalamic and spinoreticular tracts in the anterolateral white matter of the spinal cord. The spinothalamic tract (the major ascending pathway for information about pain and temperature) mainly consists of axons of neurones in laminae I and V of the dorsal horn, in which most Aδ fibres terminate. These ascend to the ventral posterior lateral nucleus of the thalamus and thence to the postcentral gyrus. Axons are somato-topically organised, with caudal elements found laterally to those from more rostral structures. The similar arrangement for mechanosensory (the major targets for mechanosensory axons are like the targets for the ascending pain and temperature axons in the ventral posterior nuclear complex) and noxious stimuli is presumably responsible for discrimina-tive aspects of pain (the ability to locate a pain and judge its intensity). The spinothalamic tract sends collateral branches to the periaqueductal grey (PAG) matter in the midbrain.[42] The spinothalamic tract is primar-ily responsible for the perception of pain intensity and localisation.

The spinoreticular pathway arises from cells deeper in the grey matter of the dorsal horn, including lamina V. Fibres ascend in the anterolateral cord and reach the nuclei of the brainstem reticular formation, from which they project to the thalamus, hypothalamus and thalamic intra-laminar nuclei.[42] The latter project diffusely to the whole cerebral cortex. This system shows little somatotopic organisation and is involved in the perception of dull, poorly localised pain impulses, the general arousal that pain causes, and the autonomic activation that follows a noxious stimulus (the classic fight or flight reaction). The cortical repre-sentation of pain is the least well documented aspect of the central path-ways for nociception. Although the thalamic neurones that relay noxious sensations via the ventral posterior nuclear complex project to the pri-mary somatic sensory cortex, ablations of the relevant regions of the par-ietal cortex do not generally alleviate chronic pain (although they impair contralateral mechanosensory perception, as expected). Perhaps this is because widespread cortical activation, mediated by projections from the central lateral nucleus and the intralaminar complex, occurs in response to a noxious stimulus. Whatever the explanation, the cortical processing of pain remains something of a mystery.

Descending modulation of pain

An extensive descending inhibitory system exists which consists of a pathway originating in the periaqueductal grey nuclei in the midbrain and descending by the raphe magnus and dorsolateral funiculus to the dorsal horn of the spinal cord, and a pathway from the locus ceruleus to the dorsal horn.

Understanding the central modulation of pain perception (on which the placebo[1.6] is presumably based) was greatly advanced by the finding that electrical or pharmacological stimulation of certain regions of the midbrain produces relief of pain. Electrical stimulation of the midbrain PAG produces profound analgesia, and during stimulation subjects are alert and their responses to non-noxious stimuli remain normal. Injection of morphine into this region produces a greater analgesic effect than at any other site in the CNS. The PAG receives input from the thalamus, hypothalamus, cortex and collaterals from the spinothalamic tract, and is therefore an important centre for descending control of pain. The PAG projects to the nucleus raphe magnus in the medulla. Axons from this nucleus descend in the dorsolateral funiculus of the spinal cord to the dorsal horn. Brainstem neurones may control nociceptive transmission by direct action on dorsal horn cells, inhibition of excitatory dorsal horn neurones and excitation of inhibitory neurones.[42] A quite ordinary example of the modulation of painful stimuli is the ability to reduce the sensation of sharp pain by activating low-threshold mechanoreceptors: if you crack your shin or stub a toe, a natural (and effective) reaction is to vigorously rub the site of injury for a minute or two. The existence of this extensive descending inhibitory system explains why cognitions, emotions and behaviour largely determine the perception of pain.

Neurotransmitters

A large number of substances are involved in pain perception, including noradrenaline, serotonin, enkephalins, β-endorphin, dynorphins, substance P, somatostatin, cholecystokinin, nitric oxide and others, and

---

1.6   A placebo is a simulated treatment (psychological or pharmacological) that is credible in appearance, but lacks a substantive, active ingredient.

knowledge of their actions forms the basis of a number of pain therapies (for a comprehensive review of the action of the various neurotransmitters, *see* Twycross[41]).

Neural plasticity

The nervous system is not hard-wired – it has the ability to change its structure and modify its function in response to the input it receives in different circumstances (i.e. it is plastic).[1.7] Plasticity is evident at all levels, from the nociceptor to the cortex. The key factors are duration of stimulation and neural sensitisation which can be peripheral (associated with inflammation) and central (secondary to peripheral sensitisation or neural injury). Peripherally, nociceptors can be sensitised[1.8] by injury, decreasing their threshold and increasing their response to noxious stimuli and becoming sensitive to non-noxious stimuli. Tissue injury is typically associated with local inflammation whereas when an axon is cut, the proximal end forms a swelling or neuroma. Neuromata may also form if a nerve is partially damaged. Spontaneous electrical activity has been demonstrated in neuromata and damaged nerves. The rate of ectopic firing is influenced by physical stimuli (heat, cold, etc.) and the metabolic and chemical environment of the nerve, and by sympathetic efferent activity.[42] Plasticity explains the recurrence of pain after permanent neurodestructive procedures such as spinothalamic tractotomy (cordotomy).

Peripheral changes are accompanied by central sensitisation. It can be shown in the dorsal horn of the cord that repetitive C-fibre activation leads to an augmented response to subsequent C-fibre input – so-called 'wind-up'. A repetitive transcutaneous stimulus to the receptive field of a C fibre in the rat leads to a dramatic (up to 20-fold) increase in the neural response in the dorsal horn. It reaches a maximum after 16 seconds and can transform 30 seconds of stimulation into several minutes of response. Central sensitisation is characterised by enhanced transmission of nociceptive information, sensitivity to non-nociceptive inputs and spontaneous impulse generation in the spinal cord. The neurochemistry of these central changes is similar to that of memory, and involves NMDA and nitric oxide. Rats demonstrate a conditioning response to the subcutaneous injection of formalin into the hind paw. Local infiltration

1.7   Plasticity is the ability of nociceptive neurones to vary their responsiveness to stimuli as a result of prolonged stimulation, chemical mediators of inflammation and neural injury.[41]

1.8   Sensitisation is a reduced pain threshold in injured tissue and the surrounding area, or in an area that is subserved by an injured peripheral nerve or an injured part of the CNS.[41]

with local anaesthetic 25 minutes after administration of subcutaneous formalin results in the abolition of sensation in the paw but the persistence of the behavioural response seen with formalin-induced pain.[43] Such observations have led to the suggestion that the memory of pain contributes to the neural sensitisation.[44] This is related to the phenomenon of somatisation that is seen in humans and has important clinical implications.

In summary, whether from a structural or functional perspective, pain is an extraordinarily complex sensory modality (recall that several details are omitted from this account). Because of the significance of warning an individual about dangerous circumstances, the mechanisms and pathways that subserve nociception are widespread and redundant. The major nociceptive pathway, like other somatic sensory modalities, comprises a three-neurone relay from periphery to cortex. This arrangement differs from the mechanosensory pathway primarily in that the central axons of dorsal root ganglion cells synapse on second-order neurones in the spinal cord, which then cross the midline and project to brainstem and thalamic nuclei in the contralateral spinal cord. The thalamic neurones, in turn, project to the same cortical areas as other somatic sensory modalities. The molecular basis of pain modulation is particularly intricate and is only beginning to be deciphered. The major features are the modulation of pain peripherally by the release of a variety of agents at the injury site, and the central modulation of afferent pain pathways by endogenous opioids that act at the level of both the spinal cord and the brainstem. Tremendous progress in understanding pain has been made in the last 25 years, and much more seems likely, given the importance of the problem.

The gate control theory of pain

The first attempt to develop an integrative model of pain designed to address the limitations of unidimensional models (such as the specificity and pattern theories) and to integrate physiological and psychological variables was the gate control theory, proposed by Melzack and his colleagues.[29,45] Melzack and Casey[45] have differentiated three systems related to the processing of nociceptive stimulation, namely sensory–discriminative, motivational–affective and cognitive–evaluative systems, all of which are postulated to contribute to the subjective experience of pain. Thus the gate control theory emphasises central nervous system (CNS) mechanisms and provides a physiological basis for the central role of psychological factors in the pain experience.

The gate control model describes the integration of peripheral stimuli with cortical variables, such as mood and anxiety, in the perception of pain. This model contradicts the notion that pain is either somatic or psychogenic, and instead postulates that both factors have either potentiating or moderating effects on pain perception. From the gate control perspective, the experience of pain is an ongoing sequence of activities that are largely reflexive in nature at the outset, but modifiable even in the earliest stages by a variety of excitatory and inhibitory influences, as well as the integration of ascending and descending CNS activity. The emphasis of Melzack and his colleagues[29,45] on the modulation of inputs in the dorsal horn of the spinal cord and the dynamic role of the brain in pain processes and perception has resulted in the integration of psychological variables (e.g. cognitions, emotions) into current research on and therapy of pain. Prior to this formulation, psychological processes were largely dismissed as reactions to pain.

The physiological details of the gate control model have been challenged, and it has been suggested that the model is incomplete.[46,47] As additional knowledge has been gathered since the original formulation in 1965, specific mechanisms have been disputed and have required revision and reformulation.[46,48] However, this theory has had enormous heuristic value in stimulating further research on the basic science of pain mechanisms. It has also given rise to new clinical treatments, including neurophysiologically based procedures (e.g. neural stimulation techniques[49]), pharmacological advances,[50] behavioural treatments,[51] and interventions targeting modification of attentional and perceptual processes involved in the pain experience.[52]

Pain in children

In the last few years considerable scientific interest has focused on the special problems of infants, children and adolescents with important implications for the comprehension, assessment and management of paediatric pain. The myths underlying past treatment of children's pain[1.9] have been refuted (*see* Box 1.3) and proved to have no empirical support.[56,57] The notion that infants and children are less capable of feeling, remembering and reporting pain has been extensively investigated by researchers and as a result there is now evidence that pain perception in

---

1.9   Comprehensive summaries of these myths are provided by Burr,[53] Eland[54] and Hawley.[55]

Box 1.3: Common misconceptions about paediatric pain

- Infants and very young children cannot feel pain because their nervous system is immature.
- Children do not feel as much pain as adults do in the same condition.
- Active children are not in pain.
- Children always report their pain.
- Children cannot reliably describe and/or locate their pain.
- Children cry because they are distressed, not because they are in pain.
- Parents are reliable sources of information about their child's pain.
- Analgesic drugs are not safe for use in children.
- Psychological interventions such as hypnosis and cognitive therapy are not effective in reducing pain intensity. They are most effective as coping strategies.

---

infants is not dependent on the degree of myelination, that pain pathways are formed before birth,[58,59] and that neonates and infants can remember pain.[60,61] Also, the child's ability to report pain from as early as 3 years of age has been supported by numerous research studies.[62–65] However, according to McGrath one of the most remarkable advances, because of its important implications for pain management, has been the gradual realisation that children's nociceptive systems are plastic: 'Like adults, children can experience pain without tissue damage, can sustain tissue damage without experiencing pain, and can experience different types of pain from the same tissue damage at different points in time'.[65]

The cognitive model of paediatric pain

Pain perception is, to a large extent, a cognitive process that is influenced by physiological, neurochemical, contextual, emotional, behavioural and spiritual variables (*see* Box 1.4). Indeed, cognitive factors affect pain perception at all ascending neural levels of pain transmission, from nociceptor input through thalamic to cortical pathways. Because the

---

Box 1.4: The cognitive model of paediatric pain

Children are not passive respondents to physical sensation, but rather they appraise their conditions.

---

perception of pain consists of three basic dimensions, namely sensory–
discriminative, cognitive–evaluative and motivational–affective,[66] the
pain experience is affected by the interaction of the cognitive and discriminative dimensions through which pain is sensed and perceived
(i.e. the sensory–discriminative dimension), the primary cognitive constructs by means of which pain is evaluated and its implications are
appraised (i.e. the cognitive–evaluative dimension), and the motivational variables that affect the emotional reactions of the individual
who is in pain (i.e. the motivational–affective dimension).

The role of cognition, emotion, behaviour, physiology and context

Although a noxious stimulus initiates a sequence of neural events many
variables intervene to modify nociception and determine the actual pain
sensation, as illustrated in Figure 1.4, perceived/experienced by an individual.[1.10] (For a cognitive-behavioural approach to paediatric pain see
McGrath.[65]) Some *individual-specific* variables, such as age, gender,
developmental level and previous pain experience, filter the way children interpret the various sensations that are caused by a noxious stimulus. Moreover, cognitive, behavioural, physiological and emotional
variables also affect the pain sensation. All these interacting variables
represent a unique, dynamic combination between the child experiencing pain and the context in which the pain is experienced.[65,67] These
factors will be briefly discussed below.

Cognitive factors are the children's thoughts and mental images
regarding pain and include appraisals both of the situation and the child's
coping resources and expectations (the pain will last for ever vs. it is time
limited, attitudes [I am helpless], visual images [a huge needle] and
beliefs). Young cancer patients evidence several important categories of
pain beliefs, including the causes of pain (mysterious vs. explainable), its
consequences (manageable vs. overwhelming and catastrophic), its temporal pattern and intensity (variable in severity vs. constantly severe),
and its locus of responsibility (patient vs. doctors vs. chance). Certain
beliefs in each of these categories are associated with anxiety, depression
and poor responses to coping efforts. Beliefs about oneself in relation to
others and the world mediate responses such as alienation, hostility and

---

1.10   Nociception can be defined as the activity produced in the nervous system by poten-
       tially tissue-damaging stimuli. Nociception may or may not be accompanied by
       pain. Thus pain is not equivalent to nociception, but rather it is best conceptualised
       as the *perception* of nociception.

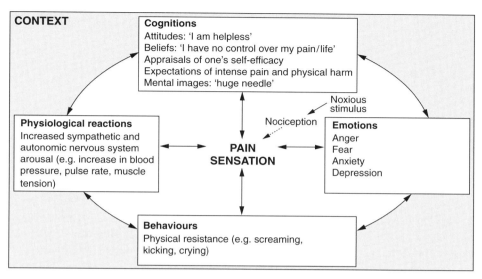

Figure 1.4:   The cognitive model of paediatric pain. Adapted from Liossi C (1999) Management of paediatric procedure related cancer pain. *Pain Rev.* 6: 279–302.

either adherence or non-adherence to pain management and even cancer treatment in general.[67,69-71]

Patients' interpretations of nociception and their resources can have both direct and indirect effects on physiological processes that may exacerbate pain. Cognitive interpretations may have a direct effect on physiology by increasing autonomic and sympathetic nervous system arousal and, potentially, muscle spasm.[72,73] Several mechanisms may account for the influence of cognitive variables on pain perception and patients' responses to treatment. Some research has suggested that there is a *direct* effect of cognition on physiology. Flor and colleagues[73] reported that thinking about stress and pain resulted in increased muscular arousal at the specific site of pain for a subset of patients with low back pain. Bandura and his colleagues reported the direct effects of self-efficacy beliefs on stress hormones[72] and levels of endorphins.[72]

Behavioural factors include children's verbal and non-verbal behaviours before, during and after the occurrence of pain. Behaviours can be adaptive and functional, and facilitate the procedure or the recovery from pain (e.g. relaxing the body, assuming the correct position) or maladaptive and dysfunctional, contributing to the child's suffering (e.g. screaming, fighting).[65,74-76] Behaviours are determined by cognitions, emotions and physiological arousal and, in turn, to a great extent determine emotions, cognitions and physiological responses.

Emotion is an individual reaction to a salient event, characterised by physiological, experiential and overt behavioural change. The same event may elicit different emotional reactions (or none) in different people or even in the same person at different points in time or in different contexts. Thus it is not the event but the person's *evaluation* of that event which leads to the particular emotion. The terms 'individual', 'salient' and 'evaluation' all imply a cognitive emphasis in this position. Emotion (affect) and cognition are 'non-dissociable'[77] – that is, they cannot be separated. Emotional development and cognitive development are two different aspects of the same process of the person–environment transaction. Emotion and cognition are mutually influential in an ongoing way. This is yet another reason why the management of pain in children is of paramount importance. We are in essence intervening to normalise the emotional and cognitive development of those children whom we help to undergo procedures without feeling pain and distress.

Children's emotions affect (and are being affected by) their cognitive comprehension, their ability to cope, their behavioural responses and their physiological reactions. In general, the more emotionally distressed children become, the stronger the pain that they experience and vice versa.

Physiological responses to painful stimuli are manifested as an acute increase in heart rate, blood pressure and intracranial pressure, together with decreases in arterial oxygen saturation and skin blood flow. Physiological responses intensify fear and anxiety and elicit negative cognitions. In turn, negative emotions and cognitions further exacerbate physiological reactions.

Finally, children do not experience pain in a vacuum – therefore contextual variables are of paramount importance in understanding paediatric pain. Contextual variables are both *general* and *child specific*. The *general* variables include the broad social, financial, cultural, historical and political situation.

The *specific* variables include:

- the hospital where the child receives treatment (specialised vs. general, adult vs. paediatric, high rating vs. low rating in the healthcare 'league tables')
- the treatment room (child vs. non-child friendly)
- the experience and training of the professional administering the procedure
- parents' and health professionals' behaviours, emotions and cognitions (which are directly and indirectly communicated to the child)
- the prognosis and stage of the disease (good vs. poor prognosis, remission vs. relapse)
- the purpose of the procedure (diagnostic vs. therapeutic).

In conclusion, there are dynamic interactions between cognitive, behavioural, emotional, physiological factors and context and pain perception.[65]

Implications for assessment and treatment

Although the relationship between a noxious stimulus and a pain sensation appears to be direct, children's cognitions, behaviours, emotions and physiological reactions, and the context in which the pain is experienced, all affect an individual's actual pain sensation. For comprehensive pain assessment and treatment it is therefore imperative that all these variables are identified, evaluated and addressed adequately. A further significant implication of this model is that due to the close relationship and interaction among the variables, health professionals can address the child's specific pain problem and trigger a positive chain reaction that will decrease the child's pain.

Children's understanding of pain

Developmental level influences children's understanding of and responses to medical procedures. From as early as 18 months of age, children have some concept of pain. Using story-telling and play tasks, research has shown that children are able to locate pain and suggest pain-relieving strategies such as hugs or medicine. Ross and Ross[56] interviewed 994 children aged between 5 and 12 years. These children were asked to define what they meant by pain, to describe different causes of pain and to explain the potential purpose of pain as a warning signal. Ross and Ross[56] specifically noted that it was not possible to categorise the children's responses in terms of Piaget's three stages of cognitive development. There were no age or gender differences in the children's reports. This is one of the few studies of children's beliefs about health or illness concepts which has not reported that beliefs progress through a series of stages.[78] Table 1.1 summarises how children perceive pain at each of Piaget's stages of cognitive development.

It should be emphasised that research in the Piagetian tradition, focusing on what children *do not* know, often misses out on what children actually *do* understand. Children are active participants within

Table 1.1:   Children's perception of pain

Piaget's developmental stage	Perception of pain
Pre-operational (2–7 years)	Pain is primarily a physical experience Pain can disappear magically No distinction between cause and effect of pain Pain is often perceived as punishment
Concrete operational (7–11 years)	Relates to pain physically Pain location can be identified Fear of bodily harm as a consequence of increased awareness of body 'physiology' Death awareness
Formal operational (12 years and above)	Beginning of abstract reasoning Recognition of the implications of pain Coping mechanisms not yet fully developed

their own cultural world, and comparing culturally and socially relevant concepts such as health, illness and pain with the more abstract concepts of space or time may be arbitrary and misleading.

Children's spontaneous strategies for coping with pain

The understanding of children's pain experiences has increased markedly in the past few years. However, less is known about the strategies that children are able to use spontaneously (i.e. before professional intervention) in their attempt to alter either the pain-producing situation or their own experience of pain. The investigation of children's spontaneous strategies for coping with pain is important for several reasons. First, if knowledge about children's own ways of coping is deficient, then researchers and clinicians must base their investigation and treatment of pain in children on their knowledge of adults. Thus developmental issues may be overlooked.[79] Children may use different strategies to adults in order to cope with pain. In fact, there is evidence for age/developmental differences in the types of strategies that children are capable of using.[80] Secondly, strategies that are most effective for children may differ from those that have been shown to be effective for adults. Furthermore, investigation of children's spontaneous coping strategies may have important implications for the identification of ineffective copers.

Methods of assessing children's spontaneous coping strategies have progressed over the past few years from case study information[81] to questions about coping included in more general paediatric pain interviews and questionnaires,[56,82,83] self-reported strategies elicited by imaginally reconstructed pain situations,[84,85] and most recently *in-vivo* assessment of strategies.[80,86] Peterson and Crowson[85] asked children to participate in four role plays designed to assess what the children themselves would do and what they would suggest a friend should do when encountering a medical procedure and a minor injury. Open-ended responses were coded into an empirically derived continuum from proactive coping (e.g. imagine you are somewhere else, pay attention to your breathing, try to relax your muscles) to neutral coping (e.g. sit still, be quiet, do what the nurse says) to reactive coping (e.g. yell, cry, hit the doctor). Similar responses were given for coping with medical procedures and injuries. However, children suggested more reactive coping strategies (e.g. cry, pull away) for themselves and more proactive responses (e.g. think of something that is fun to do, take deep breaths) for friends. This finding questions the assumption that children choose the most effective coping strategy in their repertoire when they themselves confront an aversive stimulus, and suggests that preparation for invasive procedures should include motivational components. These results may appear counter-intuitive, but they are consistent with adult behaviours. Adults recognise adaptive coping techniques for dealing with stress, such as relaxation and regular exercise, and recommend them to friends, yet they themselves often continue to engage in harmful behaviours such as smoking and the abuse of alcohol and other drugs. This study clearly demonstrates that children in middle childhood are aware of the types of proactive coping skills that are taught in intervention studies on coping (e.g. relaxation, use of imagery, etc.), but none the less choose to engage in less efficacious behaviours when experiencing medical procedures and minor injuries (painful or not). One reason for relying on more reactive responses may be a motivational deficit. Although children have a knowledge of classical coping skills, they may believe that the techniques are difficult to perform and therefore revert to more reactive processes. Another reason may be that proactive coping behaviours do not serve to draw attention to the child's distress. Children often look to adults, especially parents, to alleviate their distress, and reactive behaviours such as making a noise and complaining may elicit attention from adults, and thereby be reinforced. Scientists have suggested that this motivational component may be one reason why children appear to be more distressed when their parents are present than when they are absent during invasive procedures.[87,88]

Long-term consequences of suboptimal procedure-related pain management

Children whose pain is not managed adequately lack sufficient coping skills and display high levels of distress in medical situations. They may experience enduring negative consequences,[67] such as developing avoidant attitudes to healthcare.[89] In turn, these negative attitudes may influence the likelihood of seeking necessary healthcare later in life. Pate and colleagues[90] investigated the effects of childhood medical experiences and temperament on adults' medical fear, pain and coping effectiveness, and their avoidance of medical situations. The results indicated that adults' medical fear was significantly predicted by having experienced more medical fear and pain during childhood, by being more distractible, and by gender, with females being more fearful. Greater coping effectiveness in adulthood was associated with having coped better in childhood.

Those involved in children's healthcare should focus substantial efforts on decreasing pain and fear and increasing effective coping in childhood medical situations. Interventions that teach children to use effective coping skills may provide a lifetime of benefits. Coping skills and adequate pharmacological management of pain may lead to fewer conditioned aversive reactions to the medical environment, because they reduce the likelihood of pairing extreme fear and pain with medical care. As a result, less avoidance and other undesirable conditioned responses may be expected in the future. This is crucial for children with cancer and chronic conditions, because they will need to be in regular contact with medical services throughout their lives.

The following case history describes a typical procedure-related pain scenario in an adolescent.

Case history 1.1

John was a 15-year-old boy with acute myeloid leukaemia who was referred for psychological assessment and support 6 months after his initial diagnosis, with the aim of being able to cope better with painful medical procedures. John described his lumbar puncture pain as intense, sharp and agonising. He experienced it as an 'endless torture'. He stated that he could no longer bear it, but also was particularly negative about receiving general anaesthesia, as he was 'fed up with all these drugs and treatments'. He was considering stopping treatment altogether as it had been particularly stressful, including frequent painful procedures and chemotherapy courses that usually resulted in him feeling intense nausea and vomiting. He was particularly resentful about losing his hair and the fact that he had gained weight and no longer felt attractive. He was very kind towards and co-operative with medical and nursing staff, and had good relationships with other children in the ward. On psychological evaluation and discussion with the clinical psychologist, he admitted to feeling demoralised and moderately depressed. He disclosed his knowledge and awareness of his disease, poor prognosis and the possibility of death, and his fear that he might turn out to be a treatment failure. He was not discussing these issues openly with his parents, as he wanted to protect them and not worry them further, as they were already devastated by his disease. He had frequent conflicts with his father, and was regretful that his relationships with his mother and younger brother were becoming increasingly distant and stressful. He was still going to school when not in hospital, although he could not concentrate on the academic activities and he was far too debilitated to enjoy his usual athletic pursuits. There was a high level of somatic preoccupation and distress (somatisation), a mild-to-moderate level of depression but a normative level of anxiety, when compared with a paediatric cancer reference group. There was no previous history of depression or any other psychiatric problems.

On completion of the initial psychological assessment, the following key issues for psychotherapeutic consideration were identified:

- the experience of being in repeated, excruciating pain over which John felt that he had little control
- John's internalised and unexpressed anger
- mild-to-moderate symptoms of depression (e.g. concentration difficulties, loss of interest, a sense of hopelessness, decreased self-esteem, feelings of having failed, social withdrawal)
- a dearth of rewarding pleasure activities, and a marked loss of pleasure
- a strained relationship with his family, consisting of an increasingly alienated relationship with his mother and brother, and an adversarial, stressful relationship with his father
- high levels of somatisation.

This case history highlights the complex relationship between pain and other factors in conditions such as cancer that make the distinction difficult to draw. It also illustrates the psychological ramifications of pain. Psychological and physical factors, especially in a chronic life-threatening disease such as cancer, can become closely entwined and difficult to disentangle.

References

1 Cancer Research Campaign (1990) *Childhood Cancer. UK Factsheet 15.1.* Cancer Research Campaign, London.

2   Birch JM (1988) Improvements in survival from childhood cancer: results of a population-based survey over 30 years. *BMJ.* **296**: 1372–76.

3   Stiller CA and Bunch KJ (1990) Trends in survival for childhood cancer in Britain diagnosed 1971–1985. *Br J Cancer.* **62**: 806–15.

4   National Institutes of Health. *Cancer Statistics Review 1973–1987.* US Department of Health and Human Services, Washington, DC.

5   Manne S, Miller DL, Meyers P, Woolner N, Steinherz P and Redd WH (1999) Difficulties completing treatment tasks among newly diagnosed children with cancer. *Children's Health Care.* **28**: 255–76.

6   Spinetta JJ, Murphy JL, Vik PJ *et al.* (1988) Long-term adjustment in families of children with cancer. *J Psychosoc Oncol.* **6**: 179–91.

7   Daut RL and Cleeland CS (1982) The prevalence and severity of pain in cancer. *Cancer.* **50**: 1913.

8   Ljungman G, Kreuger A, Gordh T, Berg T, Sorensen S and Rawal N (1996) Treatment of pain in pediatric oncology: a Swedish nationwide survey. *Pain.* **68**: 385–94.

9   Miser AW (1993) Management of pain associated with childhood cancer. In: NL Schechter, CB Berde and M Yaster (eds) *Pain in Infants, Children and Adolescents.* Williams and Wilkins, Baltimore.

10 Tubergen DG, Gilchrist GS, O'Brien RT *et al.* (1993) Improved outcome with delayed intensification for children with acute lymphoblastic leukemia and intermediate presenting features: a Children's Cancer Group phase III trial. *J Clin Oncol.* **11**: 527–37.

11 McGrath PJ, Hsu E, Capelli M *et al.* (1993) Pain from paediatric cancer: a survey of an outpatient oncology clinic. *J Psychosoc Oncol.* **8**: 7–16.

12 Miser AW, Dothage JA, Wesley RA *et al.* (1987) The prevalence of pain in paediatric and young adult cancer populations. *Pain.* **29**: 73–83.

13 Fowler-Kerry S (1990) Adolescent oncology survivors' recollection of pain. In: DC Tyler and EJ Krane (eds) *First International Pain Symposium, Seattle, Washington, July 1988. Pediatric Pain. Vol. 15. Advances in pain research and therapy.* Raven Press Ltd, New York, 365–72.

14 Weekes DP and Savedra MC (1988) Adolescent cancer: coping with treatment-related pain. *J Pediatr Nurs.* **3**: 318–28.

15 Kazak AE, Blackall G, Himelstein B, Brophy P and Daller R (1995) Producing systemic change in pediatric practice: an intervention protocol for reducing distress during painful procedures. *Family Syst Med.* **13**: 173–85.

16 Hockenberry MJ and Bologna-Vaughn S (1985) Preparation for intrusive procedures using non-invasive techniques in children with cancer: state of the art vs. new trends. *Cancer Nurs.* **8**: 97–102.

17 Bernstein B, Schechter NL, Hickman T and Beck A (1991) Premedication for painful procedures in children: a national survey. *J Pain Symptom Manage.* **8**: 190.

18 Nahata MC, Clotz MA and Krogg EA (1985) Adverse effects of meperidine, promethazine and chlorpromazine for sedation in pediatric patients. *Clin Pediatr.* **24**: 558–60.

19 Snodgrass WR and Dodge WR (1989) Lytic/DPT cocktail: time for rational and safe alternatives. *Pediatr Clin North Am.* **36**: 1285–91.

20 Schechter NL, Berde CB and Yaster M (eds) (1993) *Pain in Infants, Children and Adolescents.* Williams and Wilkins, Baltimore, MD.

21 Hain RDW and Campbell C (2001) Invasive procedures carried out in conscious children: contrast between North American and European paediatric oncology centres. *Arch Dis Child.* **85**: 12–15.

22 Zeltzer L and LeBaron S (1982) Hypnosis and nonhypnotic techniques for the reduction of pain and anxiety during painful procedures in children and adolescents with cancer. *J Pediatrics.* **101**: 1032–5.

23 Katz E, Kellerman J and Siegel S (1980) Behavioral distress in children with cancer undergoing medical procedures: developmental considerations. *J Consult Clin Psychol.* **48**: 356–65.

24 Jay S, Ozolins M, Elliott CH and Caldwell S (1983) Assessment of children's distress during painful medical procedures. *Health Psychol.* **2**: 133–47.

25 Schechter NL, Weisman SJ, Rosenblum M *et al.* (1977) The use of oral transmucosal fentanyl citrate for painful procedures in children. *Paediatrics.* **95**: 335–9.

26 Weisman SJ, Bernstein B and Schechter NL (1998) Consequences of inadequate analgesia during painful procedures in children. *Arch Pediatr Adolesc Med.* **152**: 147–9.

27 International Association for the Study of Pain (1986) Pain terms: a current list with definitions and notes on usages. *Pain.* **3**: 216–21.

28 McCaffert M (1972) *Nursing Management of the Patient with Pain.* Lippincott, Philadelphia, PA.

29 Melzack R and Wall PD (1965) Pain mechanisms: a new theory. *Science.* **150**: 971–9.

30 Melzack R and Wall PD (1983) *The Challenge of Pain.* Basic Books, New York.

31 Collins JJ, Byrnes ME, Dunkel IJ *et al.* (2000) The measurement of symptoms in children with cancer. *Palliative Med.* **13**: 399–407.

32 Treede RD, Apkarian AV, Bromm B, Greenspan JD and Lenz FA (2000) Cortical representation of pain: functional characterization of nociceptive areas near the lateral sulcus. *Pain.* **87**: 113–9.

33 Portenoy RK, Payne D and Jacobsen P (1999) Breakthrough pain: characteristics and impact in patients with cancer pain. *Pain.* **81**: 129–34.

34 Turk DC and Melzack R (eds) (1992) *Handbook of Pain Assessment.* Guilford Press, New York.

35 Bonica JJ (1990) Definitions and taxonomy of pain. In: JJ Bonica, JD Loeser, CR Chapman and WE Fordyce (eds) *The Management of Pain. Vol 1* (2e). Lea and Febiger, Philadelphia, PA.

36 Toomey TC, Seville JL, Mann JD and Abashian SW (1995) Relationship of learned resourcefulness to measures of pain description, psychopathology and health behavior in a sample of chronic pain patients. *Clin J Pain.* **11**: 259–66.

37 Geisser ME, Robinson ME and Henson CD (1994) The Coping Strategies Questionnaire and chronic pain adjustment: a conceptual and empirical re-analysis. *Clin J Pain.* **10**: 98–106.

38 Fernandez E and Turk DC (1989) The utility of cognitive coping strategies for altering pain perception: a meta-analysis. *Pain.* **38**: 123–35.

39 Wall PD and Melzack R (1994) *Textbook of Pain* (3e). Churchill Livingstone, London.

40 Doyle D, Hanks GWC and MacDonald N (eds) (1993) *Oxford Textbook of Palliative Medicine.* Oxford University Press, Oxford.

41 Twycross R (1994) *Pain Relief in Advanced Cancer.* Churchill Livingstone, Edinburgh.

42 Stannard CF and Booth S (1998) *Churchill's Pocketbook of Pain.* Churchill Livingstone, Edinburgh.

43 Coderre TJ, Vaccarino AL and Melzack R (1990) Central nervous system plasticity in the tonic pain response to subcutaneous formalin injection. *Brain Res.* **535**: 155–8.

44 McQuay HJ and Dickenson AH (1990) Editorial: implications of nervous system plasticity for pain management. *Anesthesia.* **45**: 101–2.

45 Melzack R and Casey KL (1968) Sensory, motivational, and central control determinants of pain: a new conceptual model. In: D Kenshalo (ed.) *The Skin Senses.* Thomas, Springfield, IL, 423–4.

46 Melzack R (1991) The gate control theory 25 years later: new perspectives on phantom limb pain. In: MR Bond, JE Charlton and CJ Woolf (eds) *Proceedings of the Fifth World Congress on Pain.* Elsevier Science, Amsterdam, 9–21.

47 Price DD (1988) *Psychological and Neural Mechanisms of Pain.* Raven Press, New York.

48 Wall PD (1988) The prevention of postoperative pain. *Pain.* **33**: 289–90.

49 Catchell RJ and Turk DC (eds) (1996) *Psychological Approaches to Pain Management. A practitioner's handbook.* Guilford Press, New York.

50 Abram SE (1993) Continuous spinal anesthesia for cancer and chronic pain. *Reg Anesth.* **18 (Suppl. 6)**: 406–13.

51 Fordyce WE (1976) *Behavioral Methods for Chronic Pain and Illness.* CV Mosby, St Louis, MO.

52 Turk DC, Meichenbaum D and Genest M (1983) *Pain and Behavioral Medicine: a cognitive–behavioral perspective.* Guilford Press, New York.

53 Burr S (1987) Pain in childhood. *Nursing.* **24**: 890–5.

54 Eland J (1985) *Myths About Pain in Children.* The Candlelighters Childhood Cancer Foundation, London.

55 Hawley D (1984) Postoperative pain in children: misconceptions, descriptions and interventions. *Pediatr Nurs.* **1**: 314–21.

56 Ross DM and Ross SA (1984) The importance of type of question, psychological climate and subject set in interviewing children about pain. *Pain.* **19**: 71–9.

57 Bradshaw C and Zeanah PD (1986) Pediatric nurses' assessments of pain in children. *Pediatr Nurs.* **1**: 314–21.

58 Fitzgerald M (1993) Development of pain pathways and mechanisms. In: KJS Anand and PC McGrath (eds) *Pain in Neonates.* Elsevier, Amsterdam, 19–37.

59 Fitzgerald M and Anand KJS (1994) Developmental neuroanatomy and neurophysiology of pain. In: NL Schechter, CB Berde and M Yaster (eds) *Pain in Infants, Children and Adolescents.* Williams and Wilkins, Baltimore, MD.

60 Franck L (1986) A new method to quantitatively describe pain behavior in infants. *Nurs Res.* **35**: 28–31.

61 Grunau VE, Whitfield MF and Petrie JH (1994) Pain sensitivity and temperament in extremely low-birth-weight premature toddlers and pre-term and full-term controls. *Pain.* **58**: 341–6.

62 Abu-Saad HH, Pool H and Tulkens B (1994) Further validity testing of the Abu-Saad paediatric pain assessment tool. *J Adv Nurs.* **19**: 1063–71.

63 Beyer J, McGrath PJ and Berde CB (1990) Discordance between self-report and behavioral pain measures in children aged 3–7 years after surgery. *J Pain Symptom Manage.* **5**: 350–56.

64 Hamers JPH, Abu-Saad HH, Van Den Hout MA, Halfens RJG and Schumacher JNM (1994) Factors influencing pain assessment and intervention in children. *J Adv Nurs.* **20**: 853–60.

65 McGrath PA (1990) *Pain in Children: nature, assessment and management.* Guilford Press, New York.

66 Melzack R (1986) Neurophysiological foundations of pain. In: RA Sternbach (ed.) *The Psychology of Pain* (2e). Raven Press, New York.

67 Ross D and Ross S (1988) *Childhood Pain. Current issues, research and management.* Urban and Schwarzenberg, Baltimore, MD.

68 Liossi C (1999) Management of paediatric procedure-related cancer pain. *Pain Rev.* **6**: 279–302.

69 Peterson L and Shigetomi C (1981) The use of coping techniques to minimize anxiety in hospitalized children. *Behav Ther.* **12**: 1–14.

70 Beales JG (1983) Factors in influencing the expectation of pain among patients in a children's burn unit. *Burns.* **9**: 187–92.

71 McGrath PA (1993) Psychological aspects of pain perception. In: NL Schechter, CB Berde and M Yaster (eds) *Pain in Infants, Children and Adolescents.* Williams and Wilkins, Baltimore, MD, 39–63.

72 Bandura A, Taylor CB, Williams SL, Meffort IN and Barchas JD (1985) Catecholamine secretion as a function of perceived coping self-efficacy. *J Consult Clin Psychol.* **53**: 406–14.

73 Flor H, Turk DC and Birbaumer N (1985) Assessment of stress-related psychophysiological responses in chronic back pain patients. *J Consult Clin Psychol.* **53**: 354–64.

74 Cataldo MR, Jacobs HE and Rogers MC (1982) Behavioral/environmental considerations in pediatric inpatient care. In: DC Russo and JW Varni (eds) *Behavioral Pediatrics: research and practice.* Plenum Press, New York, 271–98.

75 Varni JW, Katz ER and Dash J (1982) Behavioral and neurochemical aspects of pediatric pain. In: DC Russo and JW Varni (eds) *Behavioral Pediatrics: research and practice.* Plenum Press, New York, 177–224.

76 McGrath PA (1994) Alleviating children's pain: a cognitive–behavioural approach. In: PD Wall and R Melzack (eds) *Textbook of Pain* (3e). Churchill Livingstone, London, 1403–18.

77 Piaget J (1962) *Play, Dreams and Imitation in Childhood.* Norton, New York.

78 Gaffney A and Dunne EA (1986) Developmental aspects of children's definitions of pain. *Pain.* **26**: 105–17.

79 Craig KD, McMahon RJ, Morison JD and Zaskow C (1984) Developmental changes in infant pain expression during immunization injections. *Soc Sci Med.* **19**: 1331–7.

80 Branson SM and Craig KD (1988) Children's spontaneous strategies for coping with pain: a review of the literature. *Can J Behav Sci.* **20**: 402–12.

81 Savedra M (1976) Coping with pain: strategies of severely burned children. *Matern Child Nurs J.* **5**: 197–203.

82 Abu-Saad H (1984) Assessing children's responses to pain. *Pain.* **19**: 163–71.

83 Jerrett MD (1985) Children and their pain experience. *Child Health Care.* **14**: 83–9.

84 Brown AL, Cane MJ and Echols CH (1986) Young children's mental models determine analogical transfer across problems with a common goal structure. *Cogn Dev.* **1**: 103–21.

85 Peterson L, Crowson J, Saldana L and Holdridge S (1999) Of needles and skinned knees: children's coping with medical procedures and minor injuries for self and other. *Health Psychol.* **18**: 197–200.

86 Smith KE, Ackerson JP, Blotcky AD and Berkow R (1990) Preferred coping style of pediatric cancer patients during invasive medical procedures. *J Psychosoc Oncol.* **8**: 59–70.

87 Gross AM, Stern RM, Levin RB, Dale J and Wojnilower DA (1983) The effect of mother–child separation on the behavior of children experiencing a diagnostic medical procedure. *J Consult Clin Psychol.* **51**: 783–5.

88 Shaw EG and Routh DK (1982) Effects of mothers' presence on children's reaction to aversive procedures. *J Pediatr Psychol.* **7**: 33–42.

89 Bush JP and Holmbeck GNJ (1987) Children's attitudes about health care: initial development of a questionnaire. *Pediatr Psychol.* **12**: 429–43.

90 Pate JT, Blount RL, Cohen LL and Smith AJ (1996) Childhood medical experience and temperament as predictors of adult functioning in medical situations. *Children's Health Care.* **25**: 281–98.

2

Paediatric procedure-related cancer pain assessment

Christina Liossi

Introduction

As a consequence of intensive research throughout the last two decades, a number of unidimensional, multidimensional and composite measures for assessing children's pain have been developed. Although the number of measures is growing, attention to the establishment of their psychometric properties and clinical utility is not. Moreover, these measures are not yet consistently used in clinical practice. Pain is a subjective, personal event that can be measured only indirectly by one of three strategies. It is agreed that the 'gold standard' for measuring pain should be what children report about their experience (self-report measures). In addition, pain can be measured by the way in which children react in response to pain (behavioural measures). Finally, the way in which children's bodies respond to pain (physiological measures) can be used.

In this chapter, the significance of assessment in pain management is emphasised and the challenge of assessing pain in children is explored. The professional, political and economic barriers to assessing pain adequately are also discussed. Key concepts of the psychometric theory are briefly reviewed before existing pain measures for infants, children and adolescents are described and evaluated. Emphasis is placed on measures that are utilised in the oncology setting.[2.1] The chapter concludes with a discussion of a proposed model of clinical assessment of the psychological dimensions of procedure-related pain.

2.1   For a comprehensive account of pain assessment in children, *see* the review by Finley and McGrath.[1]

The assessment–treatment cycle

The significance of pain assessment and measurement is based on the premise that if pain is not assessed regularly and accurately, children will suffer inadequate pain relief (*see* Box 2.1). Comprehensive clinical assessment is an absolute prerequisite for successful treatment of any pain, or indeed of any physical or psychological condition. The primary purpose of assessment is to inform the design of and guide the treatment process. Thus assessment strategies should not be restricted to pretreatment screening, but rather they should be a continuous and integral part of the treatment process. They are used to identify and target problems for intervention, to match treatments to the patient's needs and to evaluate the effectiveness of ongoing treatment (*see* Figure 2.1). The pain assessment–treatment cycle implies a reactive model of care. However, many medical and nursing procedures are known in advance to be painful, and therefore healthcare professionals should think ahead and prevent pain whenever possible.

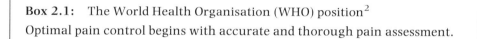

Box 2.1:   The World Health Organisation (WHO) position[2]
Optimal pain control begins with accurate and thorough pain assessment.

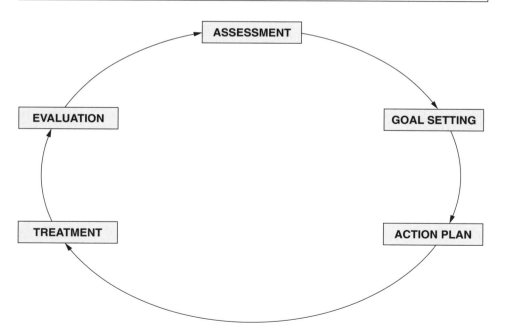

Figure 2.1:   The assessment–treatment cycle.

Children deserve optimal pain management. The first step in this endeavour is to engage in pain assessment that is reliable, valid and clinically feasible. Valid assessment of procedural pain defines the noxious impact of procedures, and determines the efficacy of pain management interventions. However, pain assessment is difficult, due to the subjective and complex nature of the phenomenon, the lack of a clear theoretical basis, the variability and inconsistency of pain expression, the persistent myths and misconceptions and, in some children, the cognitive and language limitations that may preclude comprehension and self-report.

Satisfactory pain assessment can only be achieved through professional and parental education with regard to the best assessment measures, and administrative, political and economic support for their implementation.

Barriers to pain assessment

Despite the importance of pain assessment and measurement, pain intensity measurement instruments are not regularly used in clinical practice. In Sweden in a nationwide survey[3] of 47 paediatric oncology departments, it was found that a visual analogue scale for measuring pain intensity was used in 31% of the departments and some kind of face scale was used in 23%. Systematic behavioural observation, regular contact with pain treatment teams and the use of a pain diary were rarely reported,[3] and body image pain charts and pain questionnaires were never used.

There are serious political and economic challenges that preclude patients' assessment. Low priority is frequently given to pain control in the healthcare system.[4] This is reflected in a lack of hospital policies about pain measurement in children who are at risk for pain, a lack of guidelines and quality assurance with regard to pain measurement in children, and an inadequate amount of pain education for health professionals. Economic constraints include the lack of professional time allocated to pain assessment and treatment, and failure to provide funds for specialised methods of pain measurement and management. The role of health professionals is often not clarified, and responsibility to assess and manage a child's pain adequately is diffused. All clinicians have a responsibility to provide the accepted standard of care for their patients. A clear indication that measurement of pain is a standard that must be met is provided by the guidelines for acute and cancer pain management published by the Agency for Health Care Policy and Research of the USA,[5] and the recommendations for the recognition and assessment of acute pain in children produced by the Royal College of Nursing Institute.[6] Overall, the low priority that pain has in hospitals, and the lack of education about pain in medical and nursing schools,[7] together with highly prevalent myths[8] about pain, combine to prevent adequate assessment and management of paediatric pain.

The distinction between measurement and assessment

The distinction between measurement and assessment of pain is not always clearly drawn. The measurement of any concept involves the application of a metric to a specific component. With regard to pain, measurement refers to the application of some measure of a specific aspect (usually intensity) of pain. Measurement is the quantifiable aspect of assessment and answers the question 'how much?'. The emphasis is on the quantity, extent and degree of some entity, using a standard unit. Assessment is a much broader endeavour, which encompasses the identification, detailed evaluation and measurement of the different factors of the total experience of pain and their dynamic interactions.[9]

   Although intensity of pain is clearly an important component of any assessment, many other factors contribute to an individual's subjective experience of pain. Therefore the assessment of pain covers a much broader perspective, and it attempts to account for differences in the affective response to a stimulus, the role of family styles in the perception of pain, the impact on families of having a child in pain, and the meaning of pain to the child and their family. Although some progress has been made in developing measures of intensity of pain, so far there have been few attempts to assess subjective aspects of pain such as cognitions and emotions in a standardised way.

Psychometrics of pain assessment and measurement

Psychological tests and scales are essentially an objective and standardised measure of a sample of behaviour. They are instruments designed to produce a quantitative assessment of some psychological attribute or attributes. Based on psychometric theory,[10] good psychological tests and scales should have high reliability, high validity, high discrimina-tory power and good utility. However, scales and tests may be valid or reliable in one situation or population and not in another. Therefore it is important to determine the psychometric properties of a particular measure in a situation and with a sample similar to those that are being evaluated. Some important aspects of psychometric testing are briefly reviewed below. Throughout the book, the traditional terms 'test', 'scale', and 'measure' are used almost interchangeably. Nowadays the range of psychological states and constructs that are measured is widen-ing, and the distinction between 'test', 'scale' and 'measure' may be more difficult to maintain than was the case in the past.

Administration

Psychological tests only remain reliable and valid if they are adminis-tered in accordance with the designer's instructions. Adequate training is therefore essential for the correct administration, evaluation and interpretation of any psychological test. Without such training, the indi-vidual upon whom such a test has been used may be gravely disadvan-taged, especially if decisions concerning his or her subsequent treatment are to be based, even if only in part, on the results of the test or assess-ment (e.g. provision of pain relief).

Potential problems range from the establishment of a satisfactory rap-port between the subject and the tester to the checking of the arithmetic of test marking. Improper administration lowers reliability and validity,[2.2] and consequently leads to errors in evaluation and interpretation. Never-theless, after specific short training, healthcare professionals should be capable of administering a variety of tests and scales efficiently. Training must always incorporate supervised practice in all aspects of the appropri-ate procedures. Proper administration aims to ensure that different scores reflect differences in what is being measured, and not differences in the way in which the test session was run.

Case history 2.1

A young nurse was asking a 5-year-old boy to rate his pain on a 6-point faces rating scale after a venepuncture. The senior nurse who had just performed the procedure was still in the room. The junior nurse gave the correct instructions to the child, with whom she had established a good rapport on previous occasions. To the surprise of the nurse and his mother, who had

---

2.2   These concepts will be discussed later in the chapter.

observed his distress during the procedure, the child gave a score of 0. Puzzled by this response, the nurse tried later in her supervisor's office to make sense of the discrepancy between the child's verbal rating of his pain and his obvious distress during the actual procedure, and she came up with various alternatives. One of them was the presence of the nurse who had performed the procedure during the administration of the scale. When she had finished the procedure, she said to the child 'I didn't hurt you, sweetheart, did I?'. It is obvious that the specific verbalisation and her presence altered the demand characteristics[2.3] of the situation and implicitly encouraged the child to give the 'required' response. The chances are that the patient's answer would have been different if the nurse administering the scale had waited for the senior nurse to leave the treatment room and had specifically asked her not to 'debrief' the child in this way after the procedure had been completed.

Evaluation and interpretation

It is crucial that healthcare professionals are familiar with the evaluation and interpretation procedures of a test or scale. For example, they must be aware of what a score of 3 on a visual analogue scale means in terms of suffering, and what constitutes clinical improvement.

Reliability

As used in psychometrics, the concept of test reliability covers several aspects of score consistency. In its broadest sense, test reliability indicates the extent to which individual differences in test scores are attributable to 'true' differences in the characteristics under consideration, and the extent to which they are attributable to chance errors. In more technical terms, measures of test reliability make it possible to estimate what proportion of the total variance of test scores is *error variance*. Essentially, any condition that is irrelevant to the purpose of the test represents error variance. Thus when investigators try to maintain uniform testing conditions by controlling the testing environment, instructions, time limits, rapport and other similar factors, they are reducing error variance and making the test scores more reliable. For instance, one cannot compare

2.3   Demand characteristics are the sum total of all cues available to the subject before an experiment (the experimental context), the instructions during the experiment, and the nature of the procedure itself that communicate the experimental purposes of the procedure and the desired behaviour of the subject.

pain scores on a visual analogue scale by giving different instructions to different children, or by obtaining pain measures when a doctor is present in some cases, a parent is present in some other cases or only the investigator is present in the remaining cases. However, despite optimum testing conditions, no test is a perfectly reliable instrument. Therefore every instrument should be accompanied by a statement of its reliability. Such a measure of reliability characterises the test when it is administered under standard conditions and given to individuals similar to those who constitute the normative sample.[2.4]

Since all types of reliability are concerned with the degree of consistency or agreement between two independently derived sets of scores, they can all be expressed in terms of a *correlation coefficient*. There are many types of test reliability, including test–retest, alternate form, split-half, Kuder–Richardson and Cronbach's alpha, and inter-rater reliability.

Test–retest reliability is measured by administering the test to the same group of subjects on two occasions. The two sets of scores are then correlated. The minimum acceptable correlation for test–retest reliability is 0.7. It is obvious that if anything is measured on two occasions, provided that there are no changes the measurements should be the same. Thus with precise measurement, test-retest reliability ought to be perfect – that is, a correlation of 1 should be obtained. In practice this is never the case, for the following reasons.

- Real changes may have occurred. When assessing test–retest reliability, the gap between retesting needs to be known. There may have been real changes in the variable, which affected the scores of the individuals (e.g. an increase in pain intensity).
- Other factors may produce changes. There are additional factors which can distort scores at any one time of testing, such as feeling ill, being very tired, and feeling anxious (e.g. asking a child who is upset because their mother has just left the room to score their pain).
- Test error – it is generally agreed that psychometric tests (even the best ones) measure the intended variable together with a certain amount of error.

Given the variability of pain experience from one moment to another, the reliability of pain measures can be difficult to establish. However, to the extent that an individual's average pain does not change systematically from one time point to another, then a reliable measure of average pain should demonstrate a fairly high degree of stability over these time points.

2.4   Norms are sets of scores from specified groups of subjects, and standardising a test
       involves obtaining scores from relevant groups.

Inter-rater reliability is established when two or more raters observe and assess the child's pain simultaneously.

Pain-intensity instruments for children are usually single-item scales. However, when there are multiple items which are summed to give a total score, the researcher can use indices of internal consistency such as those described below.

Split-half reliability is determined by the investigator selecting half of the items in the test at random, and calculating a total score for that half of the test, and a total score for the other half of the test. The correlation between scores on the two half tests is then calculated. A variation of the split-half reliability is *alternate-forms* reliability, in which two different versions of a test measuring the same thing are given to the same people.

Internal consistency involves determining how consistent the items are in measuring the attribute of interest. The investigator calculates the correlation (or other measure of association) between scores on each item of a test, and the total score on the test *minus* the score on the item under consideration. The established correlations indicate, for each item, how well the answers to that item relate to the answers to all of the other items.

Factor analysis

Factor analysis is a way of discovering statistical 'factors' among a large number of test items (variables). It is a way of analysing relationships between correlations, so that one can look at relationships between all variables, rather than just pairs. The first step is the construction of a correlation matrix showing the correlation between each variable and every other variable. Kline[11] describes factor analysis as a technique for finding a small number of underlying dimensions from among a larger number of variables. The final output of factor analysis includes a list of factors – which are listed in the order in which they contribute to the variance – with 'factor loadings' for each variable. These factor loadings show how much each variable contributes to the factor, and they can range from +1.0 to −1.0. The researcher names each factor by examining which variables are most heavily loaded on it.

Principal-components analysis

This yields similar results to factor analysis, but it does so in a slightly different way. Instead of looking at the relationships between variables, the principal-components analysis starts off by looking for factors which explain as much of the variance[2.5] as possible.

2.5   Variance is an index of the variability of a set of scores around their mean.

Validity

A test is regarded as valid if it measures the construct that is intended – that is, a pain scale measures pain, not depression or anxiety. The assessment of validity is a far less precise and more subjective procedure than is the case for reliability. There is no single numerical index of test validity. Fundamentally, all procedures for determining test validity are concerned with the relationships between performance on the test and other independently observable facts about the behaviour characteristics under consideration. The specific methods employed for investigating these relationships can be grouped under the following three principal categories:

- content related
- criterion related
- construct related.

Content-related validation involves the systematic examination of the test content to determine whether it covers a representative sample of the behaviour domain to be measured. Content validity is established by judgement by the test developer and content experts, who confirm that all of the relevant areas of the construct are addressed and that phenomena unrelated to the construct are not tapped. Content validity should not be confused with *face validity*. The latter is not validity in the technical sense. It refers not to what the test actually measures, but to what it appears superficially to measure. Face validity pertains to whether the test 'looks valid' to the subjects and generally to technically untrained observers. Face validity itself is a desirable feature of a test, although obviously it should never be regarded as a substitute for objectively determined validity.

Criterion validity is established when a measure is correlated with other, accepted measures of the same phenomenon. If the measure that is being evaluated is tested simultaneously with the 'gold standard', this is called *concurrent criterion validity*. If the criterion (i.e. a direct and independent measure of that which the test is designed to predict) only occurs at some time in the future, the new measure is evaluated on predicting the criterion score and is called *predictive criterion validity*. Obviously this requires there to be some benchmark measure of the variable if the correlation is to be meaningful.

Unfortunately, a significant problem with regard to determining the validity of pain measures is the lack of a single 'gold standard' with which pain measures can be compared. As a result, investigators need to consider a variety of standards with which pain measures may be compared. One standard to which all measures must be shown to hold is for the measure to be shown to be valid for the use for which it is recommended. Because a primary use of pain intensity measures is to determine the efficacy of treatment (in both research and clinical settings), one essential basic validity criterion for pain measures is that they must show change when change is expected – that is, they must show sensitivity to treatment effects.

Finally, the *construct-related validity* of a test is the extent to which that test may be said to measure a theoretical construct or trait. Construct validity involves establishing support for the underlying construct by hypothesis testing, at the same time as testing the adequacy of the measure. Construct validity is difficult to establish for pain measures in children, due to the lack of an accepted 'gold standard' or criterion measure, the paucity of reliable and valid pain measures in the absence of self-report, and the under-development of appropriate pain theories.

Discriminatory power

This is the third characteristic of good psychometric tests, and its meaning can be easily illustrated. If we were required to judge the quality of essays, it would be easy (although the actual judgements could be wrong) to put them into three groups, namely excellent, average and poor. However, these judgements have low discriminatory power, since only three groups were created, and most probably the average group would be the largest. Vernon[12] showed that nine categories are about the most that can be used with any degree of reliability or validity in any kind of rating procedure.

Utility

The utility of a measure refers to its cost-effectiveness. It involves considerations of time, feasibility and relevance to the specific clinical setting. This includes assessing the format of the measure, the number of questions, the amount of time for implementation, scoring, and interpretation, the amount of training required for its administration, and versatility. These considerations are important with regard to children, who may have limited cognitive, language, communication and attention abilities. The measure must also be relevant to both the clinician and the setting. Versatile measures have the advantage of being able to be used in several different situations (e.g. across a wide age range, or in both acute and chronic pain). For multidimensional pain measures, the health professional must feel comfortable about simultaneously communicating with the child, observing his or her behaviour, and determining changes in physiological and behavioural indicators. Utility is directly related to validity – the better the test is as a predictor, the greater are the all-round benefits to be gained from using it as an aid to clinical decision making.

The multiple dimensions of pain and the implications for pain assessment

Based on gate control and contemporary theories, a conceptualisation of pain as a multidimensional, subjective and uniquely personal experience has emerged. Multiple dimensions of pain, as discussed in Chapter 1, include the following aspects:

- physiological
- sensory
- affective
- cognitive
- behavioural
- sociocultural.

Such a conceptualisation of pain has direct implications for pain assessment and measurement. If we aim to understand and treat pain optimally, then we must assess each and every one of its dimensions comprehensively.

Pain measurement

Unidimensional and multidimensional approaches are used for measuring pain in children. Unidimensional measures may have one indicator (e.g. heart rate), one type of indicator (e.g. facial expression) or a unitary approach to pain assessment (e.g. behavioural). Multidimensional measurement is achieved by combining a variety of subjective and objective measurement approaches, or by using a composite measure. Composite measures include a variety of physiological, behavioural, sensory, affective and cognitive dimensions and contextual factors within one instrument. Multidimensional measurement is particularly appropriate when self-report is not possible (i.e. in the cases of children who have developmental, cognitive and verbal limitations, or children under 5 years of age).

Several pain measurement methods have been reported in the literature. These can be grouped into the following categories:

- self-report
- behavioural
- physiological.

A number of these methods have been extensively validated, while others are still in the development phase. A full description of all of the instruments is beyond the scope of this chapter. Instead, the tools most commonly used in research and clinical practice in paediatric oncology will be highlighted.

Self-report measures

Self-report measures are essentially the children's reports of their pain experience. They include descriptions of pain-relevant feelings, thoughts and images, and information about the quality, intensity and temporal/spatial dimensions of their pain. Self-report measures are regarded as the 'gold standard'. However, they have two major limitations. First, they require the child to have a level of cognitive development which excludes all preverbal children. Even with articulate children, measurement by self-report may be inaccurate. Young children have a relatively limited cognitive ability and may find it difficult to understand what is being asked of them during pain measurement, and to articulate descriptions of their pain. Furthermore, the current limited understanding of the developmental psychology of pain in children may prevent health professionals from asking questions in a developmentally appropriate way.[9]

The second limitation is that all self-report measures are open to bias because of the demand characteristics of the specific situation. Eland and Anderson[13] reported that, following surgery, children may deny experiencing pain when they are asked, because they fear that if they say they are in pain they will be given an injection. Ross and Ross[14] have shown that the reason given to a child for asking a question about pain, as well as the person who asks the question, make a substantial difference to the child's response. For example, if children are asked to describe pain to their mothers, they will give different answers to those they would give if they are asked to describe pain to a doctor. In addition, the type of question and the response options (e.g. open-ended vs. a check-list) may also substantially alter the child's answers.[14] Ross and Ross[15] showed that children described their pain differently to doctors, their mothers and school-friends. Clearly, demand characteristics cannot be eliminated completely from the measurement of pain. However, clinicians and researchers must be aware that a change in context can substantially influence self-reporting of pain.

The methods used to measure self-report of pain include direct questioning, pain adjective descriptors, self-rating scales and non-verbal methods.

Direct questioning

Children's spontaneous reports (e.g. 'My back hurts') or direct questioning by health professionals about pain are useful with verbal pre-schoolers and school-age children. However, reliance on spontaneous reports is likely to result in under-reported pain, as some children may not spontaneously report pain because they want to be brave, or because they do not know that anything can be done about it, or because they are afraid that they will be given an injection.

Although direct questioning is clinically useful, this approach has several limitations. Because of their unstructured nature, these methods are particularly susceptible to bias due to demand characteristics. Moreover, responses to such questions are influenced by many factors, including verbal ability, self-confidence, family variables and willingness to report symptoms. They also lack an associated measure and may be biased by inaccurate memory or the recall of a previous experience.[9]

Pain adjective descriptors

Pain adjective lists, such as the McGill Pain Questionnaire,[2.6,16] have been used successfully with older adolescents to measure the sensory, affective and evaluative dimensions of pain. A major strength of this type of scale is that it is not restricted to the intensity dimension of pain, but also measures affective and evaluative aspects of pain. Pain descriptors depend on advanced linguistic competence and therefore may not be appropriate for all children.

2.6   The McGill Pain Questionnaire is briefly described later in the chapter.

Self-rating scales

Self-rating scales of intensity of pain vary according to the type and number of anchor points provided. They may be categorised into three types, namely visual analogue scales, category rating scales and numerical rating scales.

Visual analogue scales

Visual analogue scales (VAS) consist of either a vertical or horizontal line with verbal or pictorial anchors indicating a continuum from no pain to severe pain. The VAS is a simple, robust, sensitive and reproducible instrument that enables the patient to express the severity of his or her pain in such a way that it can be given a numerical value. The most common VAS requires the patient to make a mark somewhere along a 100-mm line to indicate the amount of pain that they are experiencing. The distance of the mark from the end of the scale is then taken to represent their pain severity. Children's ratings of their pain on a VAS correlate with parents', nurses' and physicians' ratings.[17–19] Ratings on a VAS also correlate with behavioural measures of pain.[20,21] Figure 2.2 shows an example of a visual analogue scale.

The distribution of results in an unselected population of patients has been found to be uniform (i.e. there are equal numbers of measurements at all points on the line).[22] This uniformity is crucial for the sensitivity of the scale, which is one of its greatest advantages. It is difficult to measure the sensitivity of pain measurements, especially as there is no absolute standard. However, the visual analogue scale has a greater capacity to change in response to a stimulus such as treatment than the simple verbal descriptive scale, because in the latter there are not enough descriptors that can reliably be placed in ascending order of severity for pain.

Some authors[23] have suggested that a vertical scale is more appropriate than a horizontal one because children may find it easier to conceptualise the notion of greater or lesser intensity of pain in terms of up and down rather than left and right. The VAS is versatile, as it allows one to measure different dimensions, such as intensity ('How much pain do you feel?') and affect ('How anxious do you feel about the pain?').[9] However, the child must have the cognitive ability necessary to translate the pain experience into an analogue format and to understand proportionality.[9] Care must be taken when repeatedly photocopying the scale to ensure that the process does not alter the length of the line (photocopying

No pain————————————————————————————— Worst pain

Figure 2.2: Visual analogue scale.

makes the line longer) and thus confound scoring.[9] If possible, it is better to measure pain relief directly rather than to measure absolute pain on two occasions and subtract the second measurement from the first one. In the pain-intensity VAS, if a patient rates their pain at the top of the scale and then gets worse, their measurement can only remain unchanged. In the pain-relief VAS the ends are defined as 'no relief' and 'complete relief', and consequently it is impossible to be more than completely relieved. Although it is possible to become worse, the term 'no relief' is still appropriate.

Category rating scales

Category rating scales consist of a series of words along a continuum of increasing value (e.g. no pain, mild pain, medium pain, severe pain). Category rating scales may have different meanings for different children.[14] However, Wilkie and colleagues[24] have provided data which suggest that a category scale may be valid and useful for children. Figure 2.3 shows an example of a category rating scale.

Face scales, which are another form of category scale, show a series of faces that are graded in increasing intensity from 'no pain' to 'worst pain possible'. When presented with a faces scale, the child is asked to point to the face that best shows how much pain they are currently experiencing. Unlike other self-report measures, face scales are thought to be easily understood by children because they do not require the child to translate their pain experience into a numerical value. Several studies have shown that faces scales are preferred by children, parents and nurses, compared with other assessment tools, including visual analogue scales and word descriptor scales.[25–27] Acceptance of faces scales has also probably been facilitated by the importance of facial expression in the social communication of pain.[28] However, there have only been minimal efforts to validate empirically the relative merits of different faces scales.[29]

Several variants of faces scales[25,30–32] have been developed to measure children's level of pain. Despite a similar underlying conceptual basis, there are considerable differences between the various faces scales. The scales differ in format, ranging from simple line drawings,[33] to cartoon-like representations,[25] more detailed depictions of facial expressions[32] and actual photographs of children's faces.[30] Furthermore, the scales vary with regard to the number of faces that are included in the array. Some include only five faces,[34] while others include six[25] or seven[31]

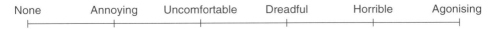

Figure 2.3:   Simple descriptive pain distress scale.

faces. The scales also vary according to whether tears are present in the 'worst pain' face[32] or not,[31] and whether the 'no pain' face is a neutral face[31] or a smiling one.[25]

There is no clear evidence that one scale is more accurate than another. The criticism has been made that faces scales which begin with a smiling 'no pain' face confound non-noxious affective states with pain – children who are not in pain are not necessarily happy.[35] Faces scales with smiling 'no pain' faces result in higher pain ratings relative to scales with neutral 'no pain' faces when used by children.[36] Although the pattern for parents is less clear, it appears that parents' ratings are also influenced by the presence of smiling 'no pain' faces. It is possible that smiling faces scales are more appropriate as measures of pain affect (i.e. the emotional aspect of pain) rather than for measuring pain intensity as they are currently used. Recent research by Goodenough and colleagues[37] examined the relationship between children's ratings on two different faces scales and a paired visual analogue method for measuring the intensity and unpleasantness of pain during blood sampling. Their results showed that the faces scale of Bieri and colleagues[31] (a neutral scale) was more strongly correlated with VAS ratings of intensity than of unpleasantness, whereas the scale of McGrath et al.[38] (the Facial Affective Scale – a smiling scale) was more strongly correlated with VAS ratings of unpleasantness than of intensity.[37] Face scales are appealing, easily understood by young children, inexpensive, and several of them have excellent psychometric characteristics. The recent proliferation of faces scales has resulted in the absence of a generally accepted version.[30] Figures 2.4, 2.5 and 2.6 depict the faces scales of Wong and Baker,[25] the Oucher,[30] and Bieri et al.[31] respectively.

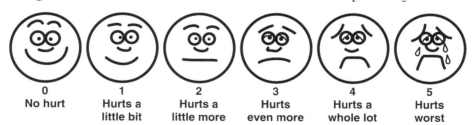

Figure 2.4:   The Wong and Baker Faces Rating Scale. (Reprinted with permission from Wong DL et al. (2001) *Essentials of Pediatric Nursing* (6e). Mosby, St Louis.)

1   Explain to the child that each face shows a person who feels happy because they have no pain (hurt, or whatever word the child uses), or who feels sad because they have some or a lot of pain.
2   Point to the appropriate face and state 'This face . . . :'
   •   'is very happy because he doesn't hurt at all'
   •   'hurts just a little bit'

OUCHER

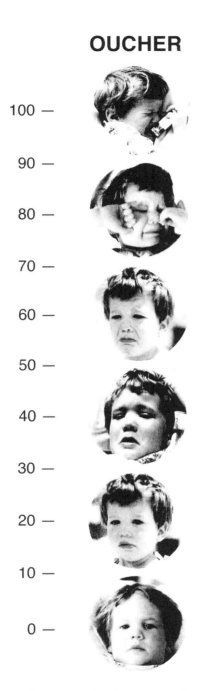

100 —

90 —

80 —

70 —

60 —

50 —

40 —

30 —

20 —

10 —

0 —

Figure 2.5: The Oucher.[30] (Reprinted with permission.)

- 'hurts a little more'
- 'hurts even more'
- 'hurts a whole lot'
- 'hurts as much as you can imagine, although you don't have to be crying to feel this bad'.

3   Ask the child to choose the face that best describes how he or she feels. Be specific about which pain (e.g. 'lumbar puncture') and what time (e.g. now, earlier before the procedure).

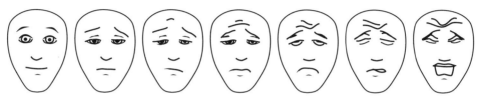

Figure 2.6:   The Faces Pain Scale. (Reprinted with permission from Bieri D *et al.* (1990) *Pain.* **41**: 139–50.)

Numerical rating scales

These scales use numbers (e.g. 0–5, 0–10 or 0–100) to represent increasing degrees of pain (*see* Figure 2.7). Children must understand number concepts in order to use this type of scale. The intervals along the scale cannot be assumed to be equal, and a change from 0 to 3 is not necessarily the same as a change from 6 to 9. Although there has not been careful work on the psychometric properties of numerical rating scales, they have a place in the clinical setting.[9] From a practical perspective, since they require no materials, are readily understood by healthcare professionals and are easy to chart, numerical scales have distinct advantages.[9] Such scales have been developed by Hester[39] and Richardson and colleagues.[40] These researchers found that responses on numerical rating scales correlate well with diary reports of behavioural and subjective components of pain. There is also good inter-rater reliability between parent and child.

Pain thermometers consist of a vertical numerical rating scale ranging from 0 to 10 or from 0 to 100, superimposed on a visual analogue scale (*see* Figure 2.8). Anchors at each endpoint indicate no hurt and most hurt possible. The child is asked to point to the place on the thermometer that represents the intensity of their pain. Scores on the pain thermometer correlate with scores on other rating scales.[41]

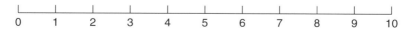

Figure 2.7:   Numerical rating scale.

Biggest hurt

No hurt

Figure 2.8:   Pain thermometer.

Poker chip tool

This tool was developed to allow children to rate their pain 'concretely' by using chips that are described as being 'pieces of hurt'. The child is able to choose the number of poker chips that best describes how much they hurt. Originally the four chips were white. However, later[42] five poker chips were used (four red ones representing pain, and one white one representing no pain). The more chips the child uses, the greater their hurt. Ross and Ross[14] have questioned the validity of the tool, and suggest that young children may not have mastered number concepts, which would make the usefulness of this tool debatable. However, they propose that using poker chips of obviously different sizes would be an appropriate modification.

Eland Colour Scale[43-45]

One of the most important aspects of this scale is that it provides information not only about the child's level of pain, but also about the location(s) of their pain. This makes it useful for non-procedure related cancer pain. The scale provides an outline figure (front and back view) with four boxes (from no pain/hurt to worst pain/hurt) for the child to colour in with their choice of colour. Eland suggests that eight crayons (yellow, orange, red, green, blue, purple, brown and black) are presented to the child, who is then encouraged to choose which colour most accurately represents the level of their pain. Once the 'key' has been created, the child is then encouraged to colour in the outlines where they hurt using the colour that is appropriate. The child is encouraged to locate the drawing with respect to time.

In summary, there is much evidence in support of the clinical utility and validity of visual analogue and numerical rating scales for measuring pain intensity.[46] These measures are intuitively simple to use, easy for most patients to comprehend, and easy to score. However, the visual and numerical rating scales and their derivatives assume that the child has the ability to reflect accurately his or her concept of pain on to a second dimension.[9] To make an assessment of pain using the visual analogue scale, the child must interpret the severity of their pain experience by identifying a point on a line where they feel that the distance between either end-point represents the intensity of their pain. Developmental psychology suggests that this metaphorical ability follows a sequence and is not acquired until the stage of concrete operations, starting at about 7 or 8 years of age. Face interval scales for measuring pain are considered to be preferable for younger (preoperational) children than more abstract scales. A scale of faces presents little cognitive complexity and metaphorical difficulty, and is relatively free of adult influences with regard to explanation and interpretations.[31]

Non-verbal methods

Non-verbal methods are used to assess the subjective component of pain. These methods include asking children to describe the colour, texture and shape of their pain, or to draw pictures of their pain. Children typically describe severe pain as being red or black.[47,48] However, red and black appear to be the preferred colours for all pain drawings, even for drawings of low intensities of pain.[48] Drawing analysis is a valuable supplementary clinical method in the assessment and treatment of paediatric cancer pain.[49] Although drawings can be reliably classified by raters[47,50] and provide valuable information about the feelings of the child towards pain, it is not clear that they can provide much information about the intensity of the child's pain.

In conclusion, self-report measures of pain are the 'gold standard' when they can be obtained. Several well-designed methods that can be easily used in clinical and research settings have been developed. However, they cannot be used with developmentally delayed or preverbal children.

Level of measurement and scales

The role of measurement scales in pain research is a complicated one, and obviously it is impossible to cover this subject in depth in the present chapter. As an alternative, the reader is provided with some basic information and referred to more specialised books.[51–53] Measurement *does*

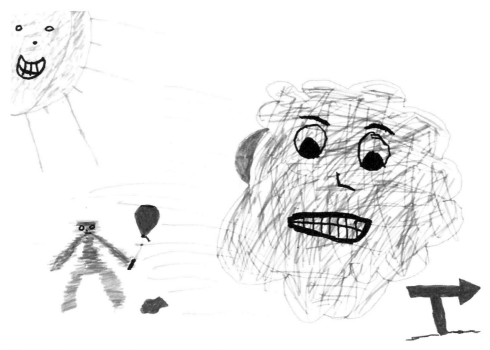

Figure 2.9:   Drawing by an 11-year-old boy with non-Hodgkin's lymphoma. It depicts his lumbar puncture pain.

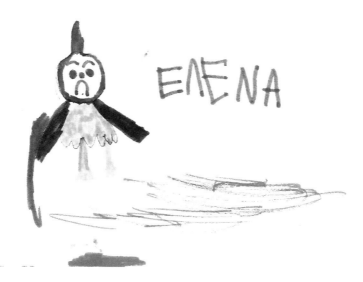

Figure 2.10:   Drawing by a 4-year-old girl with a brain tumour. It depicts her venepuncture pain.

affect the statistical analysis and the interpretation of the data that one obtains in research. There are four scales that are used to describe the measurements that we can take:

- nominal scales
- ordinal scales
- interval scales
- ratio scales.

Nominal scales are not really scales, as they do not scale items along any dimension, but rather they label them. Variables such as gender and football team affiliation are examples of nominal variables. A numerical example of a nominal scale would be the set of numbers assigned to basketball players.

The simplest true scale is an *ordinal scale*, which orders people, objects or events along a continuum. An example of such a scale would be the ranks in the army. The classification of university degrees also forms an ordinal scale. The properties of an ordinal scale are not isomorphic with the numerical system known as arithmetic. Consequently, when only the rank order of scores is known, means and standard deviations found on the scores themselves are in error or misleading to the extent that the successive intervals (distances between classes) on a scale are not equal and do not have substantive meaning. The majority of existing faces scales treat the faces as ordinal data. McGrath and colleagues[38] showed that the intervals between faces were generally not equal (that is, the perceived change in severity between faces 0 and 1, or 2 and 3, should be the same as that between faces 5 and 6). An important point about equal intervals is that they help to ensure discriminality (i.e. that two or more faces are not measuring roughly the same quantity). With equal intervals and the first face measuring zero pain, we would have the desirable properties of a ratio scale, enabling meaningful arithmetical operations to be performed on the differences, the use of the geometric mean and coefficient of variation, and the application of all of the common parametric statistics.[2.7]

The *interval scale* includes data which represent more than simply an order – it also provides information about the degree of difference between two scores. For example, if you are told the temperature, in degrees Celsius, of two different rooms, you know not only that one is warmer than the other, but also by how much. Simple numerical pain scales (e.g. 0–5) only give information about whether the pain has lessened or increased, but not about the percentage reduction or increase.

2.7   Statistics for data which conform to three parameters, namely equal-interval data, equal variance and normal distribution.

The *ratio scale*, like the interval scale, provides information about the magnitude of the differences between the entities that are measured. However, it has the additional property that the data should have a true zero (i.e. the property being measured has no quantity). For example, weight in kilograms or height in centimetres is expressed on a ratio scale. Visual analogue scales have ratio properties.[54]

Behavioural measures

Behaviour observation procedures approach the problem of pain assessment from the vantage point of behavioural indices of pain rather than pain *per se*, and so serve as useful adjuncts to the self-report procedures, physiological measures and documented tissue trauma data that are available to the clinician or researcher.[14] Behavioural pain scales record how children respond physically when they experience pain. A trained observer observes children and records any behaviours that suggest discomfort (e.g. crying). Often behaviours are assigned numbers to represent different intensities of distress.

There are three types of behaviour observation procedure that are commonly used in the assessment of paediatric pain. In *behaviour rating scales*, trained raters observe the child in a particular situation for a predetermined period of time and record the frequency of occurrence of specific, operationally defined, pain-related verbal and non-verbal behaviours. *Global rating scales* involve an observer who generally knows the child well making a single assessment about some facet of the child's pain-related behaviour during a specific procedure, such as a venepuncture, or at the end of a specific period of time. *Indirect measures of pain* focus on pain-related behaviours, such as the number of requests for medication, time spent playing out of bed, or the level of school absenteeism, and these are recorded by an observer (usually the nurse or parent).

Behavioural responses are invaluable for inferring pain in children who cannot rate their pain. The most predominant behavioural indicators of pain include facial expression, crying or vocalisation, body movement and verbal report. However, there is the challenge of distinguishing behaviour due to other forms of distress, such as hunger, thirst, anxiety, fear or loneliness, and over-stimulation from behaviour due to pain. Moreover, although these scales can provide a reliable and valid quantitative index of children's overt distress, what children do (particularly during a short observation period) does not indicate reliably how strong their pain feels. Children do not exhibit distress in direct proportion to the intensity of their pain, so pain scores on behavioural measures do not always correlate with children's own reports of pain intensity.

Some children behave stoically despite experiencing pain, whereas
others may exhibit overt distress because they are afraid or anxious.
Clinicians may misinterpret behaviours such as sleeping, watching television or using humour as the absence of pain, when in fact the child is
attempting to control his or her pain. Infants may become apathetic and
refuse to communicate after only a few days of continuous severe pain,
and suffering experienced by older children with cancer may blunt their
behaviours. Other factors that inhibit behavioural responses include
intubation, use of sedatives, the final phases of the illness, weakness
and depression. Therefore the use of behavioural observation is very
useful for guidelines, but requires close attention to the context. The
best reliability and validity of behavioural measures have been obtained
in studies of short, sharp pain such as that caused by needle procedures
(e.g. venepuncture, heelstick or lumbar punctures).[55]

Three behaviour rating scales have been developed to measure distress
in paediatric oncology patients due to bone-marrow aspirations and
lumbar punctures,[2.8] namely the Procedural Behaviour Rating Scale,[57]
the Procedure Behaviour Check-List[58] and the Observational Scale of Behavioural Distress.[59] Behaviours for observation include crying, screaming, physical restraint, verbal resistance, requests for emotional support,
muscular rigidity, verbal pain expression, flailing, nervous behaviour and
information seeking. The developers of all three scales believe that anxiety
and pain cannot be separated in the paediatric oncology patient's behaviour. No distinction can be made between behaviour that is primarily
anxiety related and pain-specific behaviour. This position has been criti-
cised because it does not distinguish, for example, between the anticipatory crying of a child in the waiting-room, which almost certainly reflects
anxiety, and the crying during the needle procedure that is due to pain.
Although anxiety exacerbates the pain experience, and pain causes anxiety, the distinction between these constructs is imperative from both theoretical and clinical perspectives. Other disadvantages of behavioural
check-lists include the fact that behavioural expressions of pain reflect a
number of individual differences which are assumed to indicate distress,
but which may be adaptive coping responses for some children, and the
fact that adolescents usually display fewer overt pain responses, and also
that observers' characteristics, such as experience and attitude, can affect
observation scores.[58]

2.8   Gauvain-Piquard et al.[56] developed a 15-item behavioural rating scale for paediatric
       oncology patients between the ages of 2 and 6 years experiencing cancer-related
       pain. The scale consists of three subscales: pain behaviours toward the affected area;
       psychomotor alterations, such as slowing down and withdrawal; and anxiety behav-
       iours, such as nervousness and irritability. The scale has adequate sensitivity
       between patients and satisfactory inter-rater reliability.

Procedural Behaviour Rating Scale

Katz and colleagues[57] developed and subsequently revised the Procedural Behaviour Rating Scale (PBRS). This instrument consists of 13 operationally defined behaviours indicative of distress which young oncology patients exhibit prior to, during and after bone-marrow aspirations. Behaviours are coded by observers for occurrence during discrete phases of medical procedures. The PBRS has an inter-rater reliability of 0.85, but there are few data on its validity. One problem specific to this scale is that it does not discriminate intensity of upset, but instead merely documents the occurrence or non-occurrence of the 13 behaviours during the aversive procedures. This means that a few tears and violent sobbing are given identical ratings, and a child who exhibits a variety of behaviours will be scored higher than one who exhibits only a few of them. The simplicity of this form of scoring generally yields high inter-rater reliability, but at the expense of the quality of information that is obtained.[14]

Procedure Behaviour Check-List

On the basis of behaviour observations and extensive interviews with paediatric leukaemia patients about their pain experience, LeBaron and Zeltzer[58] selected eight behaviours that were identical or similar to those of the PBRS to form the Procedure Behaviour Check-List (PBCL). In this adaptation, operationally defined behaviours are coded by observers for occurrence during discrete phases of the medical procedure. A major problem with the PBCL is overlapping of categories. For example, 'physical resistance' often includes 'muscle tension', and 'screaming' sometimes includes 'crying'. Since these behaviours can occur either together or independently, rater reliability can become a problem. However, in many studies the inter-rater reliability is satisfactory.[60,61]

Observational Scale of Behavioural Distress

The Observational Scale of Behavioural Distress (OSBD)[59] is a model of careful scale development. It is an 8-item modification of the PBRS that introduces two important refinements to the PBRS procedure. Behaviours are recorded at continuous 15-second intervals within each of the four phases of the medical procedure (first 3 minutes in the treatment room, first cleansing of site and Mizzy Gun, second cleansing and aspiration, removal of needle and post-procedure recovery) rather than being recorded once for occurrence or non-occurrence over an entire phase. Each of the eight behavioural categories (information seeking, crying, screaming, restraint, verbal resistance, emotional support, verbal pain and flailing) is weighted according to intensity. For example, 'nervous behaviour' is 1.0, 'verbal resistance' is 2.5 and 'screaming' is 4.0. The reliability and validity of the OSBD are satisfactory.[62,63] The OSBD is more complex than the PBRS and the PBCL, and the information that it provides is more precise.[59]

Physiological measures

A number of physiological indicators have been used to measure pain in children. Physiological indices associated with pain and anxiety include heart rate,[64] respiration rate,[65] sweating,[66] transcutaneous pO_2,[65] pulse and blood pressure.[67]

Changes in these parameters reflect a generalised and complex response to stress-inducing stimulation, rather than a specific localised response to pain intensity. Physiological methods of measuring pain provide important information about the body's response to insult, and are therefore particularly informative to the clinician, as they provide feedback on the medical stability of the child. However, care needs to be taken when using physiological measures in isolation as, after a period of time, adaptation takes place and physiological changes no longer occur.[9]

Assessment of the preverbal child

Assessment of pain in the preverbal child is extremely difficult, and these children are at particular risk for non-addressing and under-treatment of pain. Preverbal children are considered to be those who are unable to use self-report pain measures, and the category includes infants, small children, mentally handicapped and some physically handicapped children, intubated and/or paralysed children in the intensive-care unit, and children whose consciousness is impaired due to head injury or other causes. Since preverbal children cannot provide us with information about their pain, their assessment is necessarily based on behavioural and physiological measures of pain. Physiological measures that have been used with preverbal children (not necessarily in procedure-related cancer pain) include cardiovascular variables (e.g. heart rate, blood pressure, skin galvanic response and palmar sweating), respiratory variables (e.g. respiratory rate, transcutaneous oxygen tension and pulse oximetry) and metabolic and endocrine variables (e.g. adrenaline, noradrenaline, glucose and free fatty acids).[68] Behavioural measures include observing and recording behaviours such as facial expression (e.g. eye squeeze, brow contraction and open mouth), body and limb movement, and crying. Pain assessment tools available for use in neonates include the CRIES,[69] the Neonatal Infant Pain Scale,[70] and tools developed by Rushforth and Levene[71] and Haourari and colleagues.[72] Similar measures for infants and young children include the CHEOPS,[73] the Toddler Pre-school Post-operative Pain Scale (TPPPS),[74] the Nursing Assessment of Pain Intensity,[75] the Paediatric Objective Pain Score,[76] the Pain/Discomfort Score[77] and the Post-operative Pain Score.[78]

Measurement of parental distress

Remarkably few parent report measures for child distress during procedures exist in the literature. The most useful one, namely the Perception of Procedures Questionnaire,[79] is described below.

Perception of Procedures Questionnaire

The Perception of Procedures Questionnaire (PPQ) consists of 19 seven-point Likert-type questions, with lower scores indicating higher satisfaction and less distress. It is easily administered to parents (completion time is less than 10 minutes) and provides data on both child and parent distress. It assesses the immediate procedural context while also reflecting parental perceptions of general satisfaction with and involvement in their child's treatment. It has good psychometric properties. Factor analyses yielded five factors for parents, namely parent satisfaction, child distress during the procedure, child distress before the procedure, parent distress and parent involvement. Parents are asked about their communication with the healthcare team, their views of the team's commitment to parental concerns about treatment and related side-effects, the extent to which services are comprehensive and include emotional support, their perceptions of their own involvement, and their view of their child's as well as their own distress.

Pain assessment instruments

Although measurement of pain in children has become increasingly sophisticated, assessment has lagged behind. Three structured pain interviews and questionnaires have been developed for children. The Paediatric Pain Questionnaire[80] includes eight questions about the pain history, pain language, the colours that children associate with pain, the emotions which they experience, their worst pain experiences, the ways in which they cope with pain, the positive aspects of pain, and the location of their current pain.

The Varni/Thompson Paediatric Pain Questionnaire[81] is used to provide a comprehensive assessment of the child's and the parent's perception of the child's pain experience. It includes visual analogue scales, colour-coded rating scales and verbal descriptors to provide information about the sensory, affective and evaluative dimensions of children's chronic pain, as well as information about the child's and family's pain history, symptoms and pain relief interventions, and socio-environmental situations that may influence pain. It is completed separately by the child, parent and physician.

The Children's Comprehensive Pain Questionnaire (CCPQ)[82] was developed as a structured interview for children with recurrent or persistent pain. It provides information about the sensory dimensions of pain and the contributing cognitive, behavioural and emotional factors. It contains both open-ended and supplied format questions, as well as analogue rating scales, and can be used to compare pain profiles in order to evaluate new therapies.

Although they are useful as basic instruments, these questionnaires have not been guided by an explicit conceptual model.

The McGill Pain Questionnaire (MPQ)[16] can be used with older adolescents. This consists of 78 terms describing the quality and intensity of the pain. These are typically represented as 20 clusters of between three and five similar descriptors ordered from least to most painful (e.g. nagging, nauseating, agonising, dreadful and torturing). Respondents circle the descriptive clusters that correspond to their pain experience. The questionnaire has four subscales. The sensory and evaluative subscales rate the intensity and type of pain experienced. The third scale measures the emotional response to the pain, while the fourth scale captures a number of miscellaneous items. There is a short and long form, and consequently the time required to complete the questionnaire ranges from 2 to 15 minutes.

Which measure should be used?

A wide variety of unidimensional and multidimensional measures are available for assessing pain in infants and children. When selecting the most appropriate measure, the child's age, cognitive level, verbal capacity, type of pain and context (clinical and/or research) need to be considered. The quality of the measure in terms of the psychometric properties established and the purpose of assessment are also important. Finally, the clinical and research utility of the measure should be checked (e.g. length, clarity, ease of use, and time needed for use).

All of the measurement methods described above can be used either alone or in combination. There is a need to employ multiple measures in the clinical assessment of patients. Psychometric measures should be combined with clinical interviews and other methods in order to obtain the most contextually relevant picture of a patient's pain problem. Intensity scales are best suited to the assessment of acute pain and pain of short duration. Behavioural and physiological measures, when used together, can provide a more accurate picture of pain in neonates and very young infants. Multidimensional methods of pain assessment are most appropriate for assessing chronic and recurrent pain in children.

When deciding whether or not to obtain and use a particular test or scale, the healthcare professional should consider the following:

- the aims and objectives of the test
- the purpose of measurement
- the rationale for using this specific instrument for this specific measurement situation and population
- the type of research evidence cited, if any, about the measure
- the reliability of the test
- the validity of the test
- the discriminatory power of the test
- utility
- appropriate group and clinical situation.

Psychological assessment of pain

Comprehensive psychological clinical assessment of any paediatric pain, and procedure-related pain in particular, should include collection of information about the following:

- the physical and temporal qualities of the pain
- the patient's affective distress
- the patient's cognitions, such as evaluative perceptions and pain-related beliefs
- the patient's personality traits, relevant abilities, talents, interests and possible psychopathology
- the patient's family.

Individualising and tailoring treatment goals and strategies to the patient requires the assessment of all these determinants of the pain experience. This in turn facilitates systematic treatment selection and targeted therapeutic interventions. A brief description is given below of how each of these domains can be assessed, and Box 2.3 provides a concise clinical interview guide for the assessment of children who are experiencing procedure-related cancer pain. Box 2.2 gives a brief description of an assessment method that combines both qualitative and quantitative techniques proposed by Baker and Wong.[83]

Box 2.2:   The QUEST[83]

Question the child.
Use pain-rating scales.
Evaluate behaviour and physiological changes.
Secure the parents' involvement.
Take the cause of the pain into account.
Take action and evaluate the results.

Box 2.3:   Clinical interview guide to the assessment of paediatric procedure-related pain and distress

Behaviour: What do you do when you are in pain?
Affect: What emotions do you feel? Do you feel sad, angry, anxious or nervous?
Sensations: How do you experience the pain? What does it feel like? Describe the sensations.
Cognitions: What kind of thoughts do you usually have before, during and after the procedure? What do you usually tell yourself? What causes pain? What is the meaning of pain? What kinds of pictures or images flash across your mind's eye when you feel the pain?
Coping strategies: Does anything aggravate your pain, increase it or make it worse? What have you tried to do to lessen it?
Developmental history: Relationship with parents and siblings, and major childhood events. Patient's goals for therapy and their concerns.

Assessment of the physical and temporal qualities of pain

Is the pain of mild, moderate or severe intensity? How much suffering is associated with the pain? The measurement instruments described above can be utilised in the assessment of the physical and temporal qualities of pain.

Assessment of depression and anxiety

Because of the close inter-relationship between pain, depression and anxiety, it is essential to assess depression and anxiety thoroughly when evaluating a child with cancer. Increased bodily awareness (or hypersensitivity to bodily sensations), as well as cognitive symptoms of anxiety and depression, constitute major aspects of psychological disturbance, and clinicians who are attempting to alleviate procedure-related pain must be aware of their existence and severity.

Assessment of pain-related cognitions

A growing body of evidence suggests that patients' cognitions, such as beliefs and expectations about pain, the causes of pain, pain treatment, self-efficacy and coping, mediate some of the relationships between pain and the response to treatment (either pharmacological or psychological). Beliefs are personal, evaluatively loaded cognitions, assumptions or conceptions about the nature of certain things or about causal relationships between related things that are held with some degree of conviction.[84]

Although each person's cognitions are unique, their content, shape and form are influenced by sociocultural factors such as ethnicity and family background. Patients' beliefs may play a key role in determining their behaviours. Adaptive beliefs motivate compliance with medical regimens and coping behaviours that are positively reinforced by pain relief and lead to positive validation. It is crucial to know whether the child views pain as a source of punishment, or as mysterious, threatening, fearful, out of control, hopeless, or a reason to worry excessively. Because beliefs are expressed in people's behaviours, it is also important to assess relevant behaviours (e.g. coping strategies). Children's beliefs about self-efficacy and control over pain may at least partially determine their coping efforts and adjustment.

Coping is what people do to try to control, manage or tolerate stressful situations such as severe pain.[85] Numerous studies have indicated that the coping strategies of patients with pain are related to several measures of adjustment, including pain treatment outcomes. It makes intuitive sense that the particular methods which children use to deal with severe pain episodes or non-painful procedures are related to the quality of their adjustment. Therefore it is important to know what coping strategies the child has employed and his or her views of their efficacy. Categories of coping strategies include diverting attention, ignoring pain

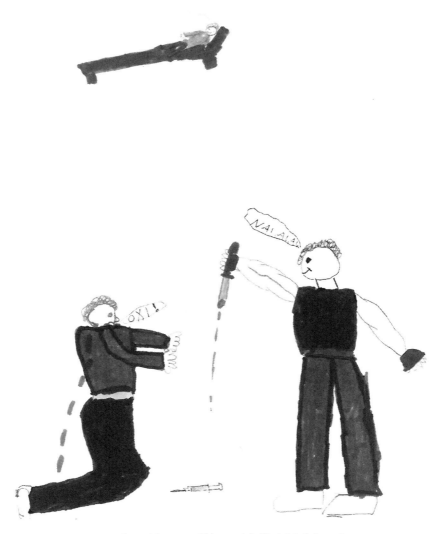

Figure 2.11: Drawing by a 12-year-old boy with Hodgkin's lymphoma.

sensation, coping self-statements, co-operating with the pharmacological management of pain, reinterpreting pain sensations, praying/hoping and catastrophising.

It is important to assess individual coping styles before planning an intervention. Most psychological interventions are based on the assumption that preparation is helpful for all children. However, some children become more distressed during preparation, and respond by closing their eyes and covering their ears in order to avoid receiving information about forthcoming stressful procedures.[15]

A useful way of assessing cognitive–affective pain responses is to undertake a cognitive–functional analysis.[86] This involves asking the child to report thoughts, images, feelings and fantasies, while imaging a stressful procedure, during the painful procedure itself, or to 'think out loud' during rehearsal. This process can be very helpful for identifying dysfunctional thoughts, misconceptions, and positive and negative coping strategies, which may then be used to plan a psychological intervention. The method may be useful for older adolescents who are able to express themselves verbally, but less useful for younger children.

Personality traits

Does the child prefer to be actively involved in his or her own care or to relinquish responsibility completely to parents and doctors? Any psychopathology or premorbid personality characteristics present should be identified and assessed. Also of importance are any talents or abilities that the child brings to the treatment situation.

The family

The child's family is paramount in ensuring that their pain experience is managed effectively. This is an important variable to assess, as parental attitudes and expectations may mediate children's perceptions and reactions.[87] Jay and colleagues[88] found that parental anxiety was one of the three variables that were most strongly predictive of children's distress during bone-marrow aspirations. Jay suggested that children who cope more effectively have parents who do not reinforce pain behaviours or display their own personal anxiety, and who are supportive and expect them to cope well.[87] Consequently, the family system should be comprehensively assessed, including collecting information about the strengths and weaknesses of the specific family, and the way in which the family deals with crises.[89] Family-centred care is important if pain is to be managed appropriately. Box 2.4 provides a parent interview guide.

Box 2.4: Parent interview guide with regard to their child's procedure-related pain

Would you like us to discuss your thoughts and feelings (unrelated to cancer and pain) at the moment?

Would you like us to discuss your thoughts and feelings related to your child's cancer and pain at the moment?

When your child hurts, what do you usually do to comfort him or her?

Which method has worked best in the past? Would you like to try it now?

Would you like to be with your child during the procedure?

Would you like to learn how you can help your child to feel less pain and anxiety during medical procedures and participate in their preparation?

The following case history demonstrates the paramount importance of comprehensive psychological assessment of a child with cancer in order to understand him or her fully.

Case history 2.2

Antonella was a 12-year-old girl with acute lymphoblastic leukaemia. She was unco-operative with medical and nursing staff, and did not make any friends in the ward. She exhibited extreme pain and anxiety during all invasive procedures, including venepunctures, lumbar punctures and bone-marrow aspirations. She was receiving general anaesthesia for the latter two procedures, but she was distressed and was refusing to fast, insisting on being given food and water before the general anaesthesia. She was behaviourally resistant during the venepunctures. Nursing and medical personnel were frustrated, and some were even resentful, that despite their best efforts this patient did not appear to respond to any of their interventions. She was referred for psychological assessment and support, which started with the aim (jointly decided with the patient) of helping her to undergo medical procedures more easily. After a comprehensive psychological assessment, the following issues emerged. Antonella's parents were quite old (which was known) and she had an older brother (who no one knew about). Her mother became pregnant unintentionally – by 'accident' as she often proclaimed even in Antonella's presence. Antonella's parents had perceived the pregnancy at a relatively older age as a social stigma, and they were feeling ostracised from the village community in which they were living. Her brother never came to visit her in the hospital, and consistently ignored her when he was visiting their parents in the village. After the disease had developed, Antonella's parents regarded her as a burden. Antonella was expressing a clear wish to die through her behaviour. She was feeling rejected, and she was perceiving her disease and the 'infinite number of procedures' as a punishment for giving her parents so much grief during her short life. She did not want to co-operate with her treatment because subconsciously she wanted to die and put an end both to her suffering and to that of her parents. The ambivalence of her feelings towards her parents was evident in that she was both punishing them (they were worried that she was suffering) and also relieving them of her presence (by trying to hasten her death). Given the complexity of her case, she received both psychological support for the procedures, to which she soon responded, and psychodynamic psychotherapy for the most fundamental psychological issues involved. Despite her good prognosis, she died a year after the initial diagnosis.

References

1 Finley GA and McGrath PJ (eds) (1998) *Measurement of Pain in Infants and Children: progress in pain research and management.* IASP Press, Seattle, WA.

2 World Health Organisation (1998) *Cancer Pain Relief and Palliative Care in Children.* World Health Organisation, Geneva.

3 Ljungman G, Kreuger A, Gordh T, Berg T, Sorensen S and Rawal N (1996) Treatment of pain in pediatric oncology: a Swedish nationwide survey. *Pain.* **68**: 385–94.

4 Twycross A (1999) Pain management: a nursing priority? *J Child Health Care.* **3**: 19–25.

5 Carr DB *et al.* (1992) *Acute Pain Management: operative or medical procedures and trauma.* Department of Health and Human Services, Rockville, MD.

6 Royal College of Nursing Institute (1999) The recognition and assessment of acute pain in children. Recommendations. In: *Pediatric Pain Sourcebook.* RCN, London.

7 Twycross A (2000) Education about pain: a neglected area? *Nurse Educ Today.* **20**: 244–53.

8 Twycross A (1998) Dispelling modern-day myths about children's pain. *J Child Health Care.* **2**: 31–5.

9 McGrath PJ and Unruh AM (1987) *Pain in Children and Adolescents.* Elsevier, Amsterdam.

10 Cronbach LJ (1970) *Essentials of Psychological Testing.* Harper and Row, New York.

11   Kline P (2000) *A Psychometrics Primer.* Free Association Books, London.

12   Vernon PE (1961) *The Measurement of Abilities.* University of London Press, London.

13   Eland JM and Anderson JE (1977) The experience of pain in children. In: A Jacox (ed.) *Pain: a source book for nurses and other professionals.* Little, Brown & Co., Boston, MA, 453–73.

14   Ross DM and Ross SA (1988) Assessment of pediatric pain: an overview. *Issues Compr Pediatr Nurs.* **11**: 73–91.

15   Ross DM and Ross SA (1984) The importance of type of question, psychological climate and subject set in interviewing children about pain. *Pain.* **19**: 71–9.

16   Melzack R (1975) The McGill Pain Questionnaire: major properties and scoring methods. *Pain.* **1**: 277–99.

17   O'Hara M, McGrath PJ, D'Astous J and Vair CA (1987) Oral morphine versus injected meperidine (Demerol) for pain relief in children after orthopaedic surgery. *J Pediatr Orthop.* **7**: 78–82.

18   Varni JW, Thompson KL and Hanson V (1987) The Varni/Thompson Pediatric Pain Questionnaire. 1. Chronic musculoskeletal pain in juvenile rheumatoid arthritis. *Pain.* **28**: 27–38.

19   McGrath PJ, Hsu E, Cappelli M *et al.* (1990) Pain from pediatric cancer: a survey of an outpatient oncology clinic. *J Psychosoc Oncol.* **8**: 109–24.

20   McGrath PJ, Johnson G, Goodman TJ *et al.* (1985) The CHEOPS: a behavioral scale to measure postoperative pain in children. In: HL Fields, R Dubner and F Cervero (eds) *Advances in Pain Research and Therapy.* Raven Press, New York.

21   Maunuksela EL, Olkkola KT and Korpela R (1987) Measurement of pain in children with self-reporting and behavioral assessment. *Clin Pharm Ther.* **42**: 137–41.

22   McGrath P, Seifert C, Speechley K, Booth J, Stitt L and Gibson M (1996) A new analogue scale for assessing children's pain: an initial validation study. *Pain.* **64**: 435–43.

23   Gaston-Johansson F (1996) Measurement of pain: the psychometric properties of the Pain-O-Meter, a simple, inexpensive pain assessment tool that could change health care practices. *J Pain Symptom Manage.* **12**: 172–81.

24   Wilkie DJ, Holzemer WL, Tesler MD *et al.* (1990) Measuring pain quality: validity and reliability of children's and adolescents' pain language. *Pain.* **41**: 151–9.

25   Wong D and Baker C (1988) Pain in children: comparison of assessment scales. *Pediatr Nurs.* **14**: 9–17.

26   West N, Oakes L, Hinds PS *et al.* (1994) Measuring pain in pediatric oncology ICU patients. *J Pediatr Oncol Nurs.* **11**: 64–8.

27 Fogel-Keck J, Gerkensmeyer JE, Joyce BA and Schade JG (1996) Reliability and validity of the faces and word descriptor scales to measure procedural pain. *J Pediatr Nurs.* **11**: 368–74.

28 Craig KD, Gilbert CA and Lilley CM (1996) Social barriers to optimal pain management in infants and children. *Clin J Pain.* **12**: 232–42.

29 Johnston CC (1998) Psychometric issues in the measurement of pain. In: GA Finley and PJ McGrath (eds) *Measurement of Pain in Infants and Children: progress in pain research and management.* IASP Press, Seattle, WA, 5–20.

30 Beyer JE (1984) *The Oucher: a user's manual and technical report.* The Hospital Play Equipment Co., Evanston, IL.

31 Bieri D, Reeve RA, Champion GD, Addicoat L and Zielger JB (1990) The faces pain scale for the self-assessment of the severity of pain experienced by children: development, initial validation, and preliminary investigation for ratio scale properties. *Pain.* **41**: 139–50.

32 Kuttner L and Lepage T (1989) Faces scales for the assessment of pediatric pain: a critical review. *Can J Behav Sci.* **21**: 198–209.

33 Maunuksela EL and Olkkola KT (1991) Pediatric pain management. *Int Anesthesiol Clin.* **29**: 37–55.

34 LeBaron S and Zeltzer L (1984) Assessment of acute pain and anxiety in children and adolescents by self-reports, observer reports and a behavior checklist. *J Consult Clin Psychol.* **52**: 729–38.

35 Champion GD, Goodenough B, von Baeyer CL and Thomas W (1998) Measurement of pain by self-report. In: GA Finley and PI McGrath (eds) *Measurement of Pain in Infants and Children: progress in pain research and management.* IASP Press, Seattle, WA, 123–60.

36 Chambers CT and Craig KD (1998) An intrusive impact of anchors in children's faces pain scales. *Pain.* **78**: 27–37.

37 Goodenough B, Champion GD, Brouwer N, Van Dongen K and Abu-Saad H (1999) *A comparison of the faces pain scale and the facial affective scale for children's self-report of pain during blood sampling procedures.* Paper presented at the 20th Annual Meeting of the Australian Pain Society.

38 McGrath PA, de Veber LL and Hearn MT (1985) Multidimensional pain assessment in children. In: HL Fields (ed.) *Advances in Pain Research and Therapy.* 9. Raven Press, New York, 387–93.

39 Hester NK (1979) The pre-operational child's reaction to immunization. *Nurs Res.* **28**: 250–5.

40 Richardson GM, McGrath P, Cunningham SJ *et al.* (1983) Validity of the headache diary for children. *Headache.* **23**: 184–7.

41 Szyfelbein SK, Osgood PF and Carr DB (1985) The assessment of pain and plasma beta-endorphin immunoactivity in burned children. *Pain.* **22**: 173–82.

42 Jakobs H and Rister M (1997) Measurement of pain in children. *Klin Paediatr.* **209**: 384–8.

43 Eland J and Anderson J (1977) The experience of pain in children. In: A Jacox (ed.) *A Source Book for Nurses and Other Health Professionals.* Little, Brown & Co., Boston, MA, 453–76.

44 Eland J (1985) The child who is hurting. *Semin Oncol Nurs.* **1**: 116–22.

45 Eland J (1990) Pain in children. *Nurs Clin North Am.* **25**: 871–4.

46 Jensen MP, Karoly P and Huger R (1987) The development and preliminary validation of an instrument to assess patients' attitudes toward pain. *J Psychosom Res.* **31**: 393–400.

47 Unruh A, McGrath PJ, Cunningham SJ *et al.* (1983) Children's drawings of their pain. *Pain.* **17**: 385–92.

48 Kurylyszyn N, McGrath PJ, Cappelli M *et al.* (1987) Children's drawings: what can they tell us about intensity of pain? *Clin J Pain.* **2**: 155–8.

49 Liossi C (2000) Understanding children's pain through drawings. *Eur J Palliative Care.* **7**: 222–5.

50 Hatira P and Liossi P (1995) Children's depiction of procedure-related cancer pain. Unpublished data.

51 Siegel S and Castellan J (1988) *Non-Parametric Statistics for the Behavioral Sciences.* McGraw-Hill, New York.

52 Hayes N (2000) *Doing Psychological Research.* Open University Press, Buckingham.

53 Howell DC (1997) *Statistical Methods for Psychology.* Duxbury Press, London.

54 Price DD, Bush FM, Long S and Harkins SW (1994) A comparison of pain measurement characteristics of mechanical visual analogue and simple numerical rating scales. *Pain.* **56**: 217–26.

55 Fradet C, McGrath PJ, Kay J *et al.* (1990) A prospective survey of reactions to blood tests by children and adolescents. *Pain.* **40**: 53–60.

56 Gauvain-Piquard A, Rodary C, Rezvani A and Lemerle J (1987) Pain in children aged 2–6 years: a new observational rating scale elaborated in a paediatric oncology unit – preliminary report. *Pain.* **31**: 177–88.

57 Katz E, Kellerman J and Siegel S (1980) Behavioural distress in children with cancer undergoing medical procedures: developmental considerations. *J Consult Clin Psychol.* **48**: 356–65.

58 LeBaron S and Zeltzer L (1984) Assessment of acute pain and anxiety in children and adolescents by self-reports, observer reports and a behaviour checklist. *J Consult Clin Psychol.* **52**: 729–38.

59 Jay SM and Elliott CH (1984) Behavioral observation scales for measuring children's distress: the effects of increased methodological rigor. *J Consult Clin Psychol.* **52**: 1106–7.

60 Hawkins PJ, Liossi C, Ewart B, Hatira P and Kosmidis H (1998) Hypnosis in the alleviation of procedure-related pain and distress in pediatric oncology patients. *Contemp Hypnosis.* **15**: 199–207.

61 Liossi C and Hatira P (1999) Clinical hypnosis versus cognitive behavioral training for pain management with pediatric cancer patients undergoing bone-marrow aspirations. *Int J Clin Exp Hypnosis.* **47**: 104–16.

62 Jay SM (1988) Invasive medical procedures. In: D Routh (ed.) *Handbook of Pediatric Psychology.* Plenum Press, New York, 401–25.

63 Jay SM, Ozolins M, Elliott CH and Caldwell S (1983) Assessment of children's distress during painful medical procedures. *Health Psychol.* **2**: 133.

64 Johnston CC and Strada ME (1986) Acute pain response in infants: a multi-dimensional description. *Pain.* **24**: 373–82.

65 Williamson PS and Williamson ML (1983) Physiologic stress reduction by a local anesthetic during newborn circumcision. *Pediatrics.* **71**: 36–40.

66 Harpin VA and Rutter N (1983) Making heel pricks less painful. *Arch Dis Child.* **58**: 226–8.

67 Jay SM, Elliott CH, Katz E and Siegel SE (1987) Cognitive–behavioural and pharmacologic interventions for children's distress during painful medical procedures. *J Consult Clin Psychol.* **55**: 860–5.

68 Tatman A and Johnson P (1998) Pain assessment in the preverbal child. In: A Twycross, A Moriarty and T Bette (eds) *Paediatric Pain Management: a multidisciplinary approach.* Radcliffe Medical Press, Oxford, 77–94.

69 Krechel SW and Bildner J (1995) CRIES: a new neonatal postoperative pain measurement score. Initial testing of validity and reliability. *Paediatr Anaesth.* **5**: 53–61.

70 Lawrence J, Alcock D, McGrath P *et al.* (1993) The development of a tool to assess neonatal pain. *Neonatal Network.* **12**: 59–65.

71 Rushforth JA and Levene MI (1994) Behavioural response to pain in healthy neonates. *Arch Dis Child.* **70**: F174–6.

72 Haouari N, Wood C, Griffiths GC *et al.* (1995) The analgesic effect of sucrose in full-term infants: a randomized controlled trial. *BMJ.* **310**: 1498–500.

73 McGrath PJ, Johnson G, Goodman JT *et al.* (1985) CHEOPS: a behavioral scale for rating postoperative pain in children. In: HL Fields (ed.) *Advances in Pain Research and Therapy.* Raven Press, New York, 395–402.

74 Tarbell SE, Cohen IT and Marsh JL (1992) The Toddler–Preschooler Postoperative Pain Scale: an observational scale for measuring postoperative pain in children aged 1–5. Preliminary report. *Pain.* **50**: 273–80.

75   Stevens B (1990) Development and testing of a pediatric pain management sheet. *Pediatr Nurs.* **16**: 543–8.

76   Hannallah RS, Broadman LM, Belman AS *et al.* (1987) Comparison of caudal and ileo-inguinal/ilio-hypogastric nerve blocks for control of post-orchido-pexy pain in pediatric ambulatory surgery. *Anaesthesia.* **66**: 832–4.

77   Barrier G, Attia J, Mayer MN *et al.* (1989) Measurement of postoperative pain and narcotic administration in infants using a new clinical scoring system. *Intensive Care Med.* **15**: S37–9.

78   Conroy JM, Othreson HB, Dorman BH *et al.* (1993) A comparison of wound instillation and caudal block for analgesia following pediatric inguinal herniorrhaphy. *J Pediatr Surg.* **28**: 565–7.

79   Kazak AE, Penati B, Waibel MK and Blackall GF (1996) The Perception of Procedures Questionnaire: psychometric properties of a brief parent report measure of procedural distress. *J Pediatr Psychol.* **21**: 195–207.

80   Tesler MD, Ward JA, Savedra MC *et al.* (1983) Developing an instrument for eliciting children's description of pain. *Percep Motor Skills.* **56**: 315–21.

81   Varni JW, Thompson KL and Hanson V (1987) The Varni/Thompson Pediatric Pain Questionnaire. 1. Chronic musculoskeletal pain in juvenile rheumatoid arthritis. *Pain.* **28**: 27–38.

82   McGrath PA (1990) *Pain in Children: nature, assessment, treatment.* Guilford Press, New York.

83   Baker C and Wong D (1987) QUEST: a process of pain assessment in children. *Orthopaed Nurs.* **6**: 9–17.

84   Turk DC, Meichenbaum D and Genest M (1983) *Pain and Behavioral Medicine: a cognitive–behavioral perspective.* Guilford Press, New York.

85   Eimer BN and Freeman A (1998) *Pain Management Psychotherapy. A practical guide.* John Wiley & Sons, Chichester.

86   Meichenbaum D and Turk D (1976) The cognitive–behavioral management of anxiety, anger and pain. In: PO Davidson (ed.) *The Behavioral Management of Anxiety, Depression and Pain.* Brunner/Mazel, New York, 1–34.

87   Jay SM (1988) Invasive medical procedures. In: D Routh (ed.) *Handbook of Pediatric Psychology.* Plenum Press, New York, 401–25.

88   Jay SM, Ozolins M, Elliott CH and Caldwell S (1983) Assessment of children's distress during painful medical procedures. *Health Psychol.* **2**: 133.

89   Liossi C, Hatira P and Mystakidou K (1997) The use of the genogram in palliative care. *Palliative Med.* **11**: 455–61.

3

The pharmacological management of paediatric procedure-related cancer pain

Richard Hain

Introduction

Why do we undertreat children in pain?

Children are like fish: they do not feel pain.

This extraordinary view was expressed in the early 1990s by a professor of paediatric haematology (now deceased) at a large tertiary referral centre in North America. As he said it, he would smile in a way that suggested that he realised that what he was saying was controversial and that he might – only might – be joking.

He may genuinely have been joking. However, the view he was expressing is one that was genuinely held for many years. Scientifically, its roots can perhaps be traced back to a study conducted in 1941,[1] which consisted of a series of short films of the response of children to being pricked by a pin. The study began with the children as newborns and continued to film them at intervals until they were 4 years old. From observation of the changing pattern of physical response to the procedure as the child developed, the authors concluded that the brain of the very young child was anatomically and physiologically incapable of experiencing pain. Even when fully awake, suggested the authors, children are as insensitive to pain as if they are deeply anaesthetised.

The present-day reader will be horrified at the idea that such a study could be considered, let alone carried out, and will rightly treat its conclusions with great scepticism. How could we ever have believed that children experienced pain less intensely than adults?

Yet the truth is that such a view is still held by many professionals practising in paediatrics today. The science is only part of the story. Healthcare professionals are adults, and as such they wish above everything to shield children from harm. When considering to what extent to protect a child from the experience of pain, the healthcare professional must balance this against the potential risk associated with the means used to provide analgesia. The damage caused to a child through the experience of pain is not easy to demonstrate. However, the damage caused by an opioid overdose or a general anaesthetic that 'goes wrong' is much more obvious. The result is that there is an inherent tendency to avoid or minimise the doses of medications that might otherwise allow effective analgesia. Scientific studies have often simply provided a means of justifying this bias.

If such studies are sometimes used to prop up the medical myth that analgesia is fundamentally something to avoid in children, they can also help to change this perception. In balancing risks against benefits, healthcare professionals need to know that effective analgesia is safe. Increasing evidence has accumulated to show that analgesic and anaesthetic drugs used frequently for paediatric oncology procedures carry little risk.[2–4] It is no longer rationally tenable to argue that the risk of a general anaesthetic or deep sedation is so high that it should not be offered to a child undergoing very invasive procedures such as bone-marrow aspiration. At the same time, scientific studies are also demonstrating that inadequately managed pain associated with procedures can have a long-term impact on children.[5–7] The question should probably no longer be 'Is there a good reason for providing deep sedation or general anaesthesia for this patient?', but rather 'Is this procedure so minor and so pain-free that the child should remain conscious through it?'.

Importance of non-pharmacological interventions

Physical symptoms can often be ameliorated using psychological methods, and in the same way drugs can have an important role in managing psychological and emotional aspects of pain. The fact that pain has a very large psychological component does not of itself imply that it always demands a psychological approach, but it does highlight the importance and potential effectiveness of these and other non-pharmacological approaches in managing some patients' pain.

Clearly we should not allow a child to experience unnecessary pain simply because they have learned how to cope with it, or because skilful practitioners can minimise the long-term psychological sequelae. Pharmacological approaches currently offer the only reliable means of abolishing pain completely. They are therefore the indispensable central plank of management of painful procedures in children. However, for many children, non-pharmacological interventions can make a significant difference to their experience of repeated and painful procedures. Psychological techniques also have a valuable role in preparing the child for more definitive measures, such as a general anaesthetic. The findings of a recent postal survey[8] suggest that as many as 10% of responding paediatric oncology centres in the UK and North America routinely use non-pharmacological techniques. The latter include distraction, imagery, relaxation, breathing exercises and hypnosis.

Psychological and pharmacological approaches are not alternatives to one another, but rather they are complementary, as each can address several aspects of the complex and multidimensional experience of pain.

Procedures involved

Before we look at the pharmacological approaches that are available for helping children through cancer-related procedures, it is worth considering just what it is children have to undergo. On average, the management of cancer in childhood lasts for between 6 months and 3 years. The early weeks and months in particular are characterised by frequent and repeated tests and the administration of powerful and toxic anticancer chemotherapeutic agents into muscles, veins and, via the spinal cord, the brain itself. As treatment progresses, an increasing proportion of chemotherapy can be given by mouth. However, even then there are multiple blood tests, lumbar punctures and needles inserted into the bones in order to assess the effectiveness of treatment.

Seven procedures are frequently performed in children with cancer. It may be helpful to consider these in order of increasing discomfort.

Finger-prick tests

Leukaemia is essentially a cancer of the blood, and the drugs used to treat leukaemia and most other forms of cancer in childhood have effects on the number and function of normal blood cells. The white cells in particular, which normally fight infection, are often severely reduced in number, leaving the child very vulnerable to life-threatening infection.

It is therefore mandatory to make frequent checks of the blood count. Fortunately, as technology has advanced, the volume of blood required for these tests has become smaller, and now one millilitre of blood may be all that is necessary. This volume may be obtained without the need to access a vein, which can be a technically difficult process that sometimes requires several attempts. Instead, a needle can be inserted into the pad of a finger or thumb, which can then be squeezed in order to obtain enough blood for the test. The blood is collected directly into the sample bottle.

The fingertips are rich in sensory nerve endings, and the process of squeezing the finger in order to obtain enough blood is not always a comfortable one. In cold weather it can be difficult to obtain enough blood without exerting prolonged pressure. However, the technique has the advantage that it is almost always possible to obtain a sample first time, and on the whole the finger-prick is an effective and relatively pain-free procedure. It probably represents the least degree of intervention for which pharmacological management could be considered necessary. Such management would usually constitute the application of topical anaesthetic cream (see below).

Venepuncture

Access to the veins via a needle is frequently necessary. Blood is taken by means of a metal needle that is inserted through the skin and into the vein. The choice of a vein from which to take blood is both important and challenging. Generally speaking, the most accessible veins are those in the antecubital fossa of the arm. In a warm child who is not resisting and who is beyond infancy, this procedure can be quite straightforward, and it is usual to obtain a blood sample first time. Unfortunately, most children who need blood to be taken from a vein do not fall within this category, with the result that several attempts are often necessary. Furthermore, after repeated venepunctures, the veins become bruised and thrombosed and it is no longer possible to take blood from them.

Topical anaesthetic cream can provide effective superficial analgesia. However, the veins themselves are also sensitive to pain, and although the skin can be anaesthetised in this way, the vein itself cannot. Furthermore, the cream can cause the veins to constrict so that they become difficult or impossible to access. It is rarely possible to make more than one attempt on the same vein. Since anaesthetic creams need to be applied 45 minutes before the procedure takes place, in practical terms it is very difficult to ensure that every vein that may need to have a needle inserted into it has been adequately anaesthetised.

When drugs are to be infused intravenously, it is commonly necessary to cannulate the vein. This involves inserting a soft plastic cannula using a thin flexible metal stylet. The procedure has all the problems associated with accessing the vein using a needle, and also introduces some additional difficulties of its own. The cannula is long, and veins that are suitable for taking blood may be short and therefore not equally suitable for cannulation. Because the cannula needs to be fed into the vein, this procedure is technically much more difficult to perform, particularly in small children. It is not uncommon for the cannula, having entered the vein, to leave it again, causing a large bruise and rendering a second attempt impossible. Insertion of an intravenous cannula is extremely painful even for an adult who is able to sit still during the procedure. It is usual for a young child to need to be restrained physically by one or more parents or nurses in order for the procedure to be performed.

Topical anaesthetic creams can again help to alleviate the discomfort associated with venous cannulation, and injected local anaesthetic can potentially render the procedure virtually pain-free. These approaches both have the disadvantage of making the cannulation technically more difficult, thus increasing the risk both of multiple attempts and of damaging the veins so that they cannot be cannulated again for many days.

Accessing central venous lines

Because of the importance of venous access on the one hand and the difficulty of inserting needles and cannulae on the other, children with cancer will usually be offered a semi-permanent alternative known as a central venous line. A soft plastic tube is inserted surgically into one of the major veins, usually through a smaller vein in the neck and into the superior vena cava as it enters the heart. Because the presence of such a tube sprouting from the neck would be uncomfortable for most patients, the other end is tunnelled underneath the skin of the chest. The tube can then be brought out of the skin at a convenient site, usually on the front of the chest. The protruding end terminates in a plastic screw thread to which a cap can be fixed. This can be removed when required, and the tube attached simply and painlessly to an infusion set. Blood samples can be withdrawn from the same line, so that the need for venepunctures is kept to a working minimum. This approach to venous access has the advantage of being entirely pain-free. However, there is a small but definite risk that infection can enter the line itself or, more commonly, the skin around the exit site on the chest. Furthermore, children with this type of venous access are not able to go swimming until it has been surgically removed, and the line is difficult to conceal for cosmetic purposes.

An alternative is to enclose the end of the central line under the skin of the chest. This is done by implanting a small metal box about 2 cm square with a thick plastic front. It is buried beneath the skin, but is easily locatable by palpation. For it to be accessed, a dedicated needle must be inserted through the overlying skin and the plastic front, so that its tip lies within the blood. In effect, such a port creates an artificial vein that is easy both to locate and to access. A further advantage is that anaesthetic cream can be applied well before the procedure, in the certainty that it will be possible to access the vein first time. Some surgeons, when implanting the port, will deliberately sever some of the cutaneous nerves so that the patch of skin overlying the port is permanently numb.

From the procedural point of view, the disadvantages of this approach are that a needle is still required. There is also, of course, the small but real chance that it may not be possible to access the port first time. In addition, it is cosmetically unacceptable for some children and/or their parents.

Accessing a central line without a needle clearly does not require analgesia, since the procedure is entirely pain-free. Accessing the port is more unpleasant, and indeed for some children it is surprisingly traumatic. For most, however, it too is a relatively minor procedure that requires little more than topical anaesthetic cream and good management of the attendant anxiety.

Radiotherapy

The management of many childhood cancers includes radiation therapy. The process of receiving radiation is painless. However, in order to minimise the toxicity associated with it, radiotherapy has to be very precisely targeted. This requires the child to remain absolutely still, not only for the radiation itself but also while the exact field and dose of the radiation are being planned. The whole process can take some time and several visits.

Radiation to the head and neck is particularly challenging. It is especially important for the radiation to be precisely targeted to the area that requires it, so that normal brain tissue is involved as little as possible. To this end, a plastic mask is made so that the child is immobilised in the appropriate position on each occasion when radiation is given. This can be a very frightening experience for the child, who has to lie perfectly still while something is placed over his or her face. It is therefore usual for such procedures to be performed under general anaesthetic, particularly for very young children. Although non-pharmacological measures such as hypnosis[9] have been evaluated, general anaesthesia remains the rule.

Lumbar puncture

Some cancers of childhood, particularly leukaemia, can spread into the brain, where it can be difficult to treat them. It is important first to know that the disease is there, and secondly to give treatment to eradicate or prevent it. Achieving these objectives requires a needle to be inserted into the cerebrospinal fluid (CSF) that surrounds the brain, through which CSF can be withdrawn or chemotherapy administered. This would be impossible in most children if the only place from which the fluid could be collected was within the brain itself. Fortunately, the fluid circulates not only around the brain but also down the spinal cord as far as the lumbar vertebrae at the base of the spine. A needle inserted between the vertebrae in this region allows cerebrospinal fluid to be withdrawn for diagnostic purposes, and also for therapeutic medication to be administered directly into the central nervous system. The insertion of a needle in this way is known as a lumbar puncture.

Despite its apparent complexity, lumbar puncture is a rather easier procedure to perform in most children than venepuncture. Although there is always the possibility that the procedure will need to be repeated, in experienced hands this is unlikely. The needle passes through the very sensitive skin of the back, through a ligament which traverses the vertebrae, and into the cerebrospinal fluid. The procedure is probably little more painful physically than venepuncture. Furthermore, there are fewer problems with using local anaesthetic, and injection of local anaesthetic agents (see below) is usual if the procedure is to be performed in a conscious patient.

However, although the physical element of pain in lumbar puncture is relatively minor, the procedure itself is one of the more unpleasant ones that children with cancer have to endure. In order to make the space between the vertebrae accessible, the child needs to be bent round and held tightly in this uncomfortable and vulnerable position. The child's head is buried in his or her chest so that it is difficult to cry out and sometimes even to breathe easily. The child cannot look round and therefore cannot see what is being done or even what is going on elsewhere in the room. In addition to these feelings of claustrophobia, helplessness and fear, the child is often humiliated by the exposure of his or her back and buttocks to people who cannot be seen.

Lumbar puncture is therefore not the trivial procedure that it might at first appear to be. The emotional and psychological aspects of the procedure mean that for many children it is an extremely traumatic experience. Ideally it should be performed under general anaesthetic or deep sedation, perhaps when these are being administered for other reasons. If such measures are not available, then effective sedation, anxiolysis and amnesia should be offered using both pharmacological and non-pharmacological methods.

Bone-marrow aspiration and trephine (biopsy)

Bone-marrow aspiration and trephine (or biopsy; see below) are two of the most unpleasant procedures that children with cancer have to undergo. The gap between the physician's perception of a procedure and the child's own experience of it is perhaps never greater than in bone-marrow interventions.

The purpose of bone-marrow aspiration is to draw off samples of the blood which flows through the centre of the bones. This blood is rich in the cells that ultimately develop into blood cells. It is these cells that become cancerous in leukaemia, and bone-marrow aspiration is an essential part of the diagnosis and monitoring of children with this condition. It is also performed in patients with some other cancers in which tumour cells can spread into the bone marrow.

Bone-marrow aspiration is performed from one of the most accessible bones – in children usually the posterior superior iliac spine behind the hip. It is performed using a large metal needle which has to be strong enough to pass through bone. The needle is first pushed through the skin. Sometimes it is too large to go through the skin on its own, and a small skin cut is made to accommodate it using a blade. The needle is next pushed through the periosteum (the very sensitive internal 'skin' which covers the bone), and then pushed through until it comes up against the bone itself. Finally, it is pushed hard through the bone cortex until it crunches through and the tip of the needle is in the liquid marrow itself. The marrow is then withdrawn through the needle. Even this is painful as, like the periosteum, the marrow cavity is very sensitive to pain. Bone pain due to expansion of the marrow is a common presenting feature of leukaemia. Adult patients who have had to undergo bone-marrow aspiration while conscious have described quite severe pain as the marrow is withdrawn.

It is not possible to obtain adequate analgesia for this procedure using local anaesthetic alone. Topical anaesthetic creams may be sufficient for anaesthetising the skin. Injected local anaesthetic, provided that both the skin and the periosteum are infiltrated, can be very helpful. However, it is not possible to give complete pain relief for this procedure unless the patient is anaesthetised or deeply sedated. In the UK it would be very unusual for bone-marrow aspiration to be performed in a conscious child.

Bone-marrow trephine is even more invasive. The purpose of a bone-marrow trephine is to obtain a core of tissue containing a section of the bone. At the top of the core is the periosteum, then the bone cortex and lastly the honeycomb-like matrix containing bone marrow. Trephine is performed when it is necessary to examine not only the marrow but also the architecture of the bone itself. An example would be in neuroblastoma or some lymphomas, where it is important to be as certain as possible that there has been no infiltration.

In order to obtain a core of tissue, a large hollow needle is inserted through both the skin and the bone. Again the skin may need to be incised first to allow the needle to pass through. The hollow needle is screwed 10 or 20 times into the bone and through the cortex, until it is lodged firmly in the marrow. In order to break off the core, the needle is then waggled to and fro several times before being withdrawn carefully so that the core is not lost in the process. It is not unusual for this procedure to need to be repeated, particularly in inexperienced hands.

Once again it is difficult, if not impossible, to administer enough local anaesthetic to render this procedure pain-free. Even if it were so, the attendant anxiety and discomfort could not be adequately managed. Again, in the UK this procedure is rarely performed in a conscious paediatric patient.

What does a child experience?

Holistic nature of pain

In children as in adults, pain is a complex multidimensional phenomenon.[7] The extent of actual tissue damage only correlates poorly with the severity of pain. This physical dimension must be considered in the light of emotional, psychological and even existential or spiritual issues.

Pain which occurs in the context of anxiety and uncertainty, and perhaps above all a sense of loss of control, is much more severe than pain which occurs, for example, during a game of football. In addition to the emotional components of the pain, there is an element of existential understanding. A child may never articulate the question 'What does this pain signify?', but the underlying question will always be there. If the answer is unwelcome or uncertain, the experience of pain will be more extreme. Even to a child, growing pains have quite a different meaning to bone pain due to leukaemia, despite the fact that the nature and intensity of the pain are very similar.

As has already been noted, interventions in childhood cancer are characterised by a number of emotional and psychological associations which make them extremely painful, often apparently out of all proportion to the invasiveness of the procedures themselves. They occur at a time of severe anxiety, not only for the child but also for the mother, father and siblings. The procedures are poorly understood by the child and his or her family, as there is often little time to explain fully what is about to happen, and the gap between lay understanding of childhood cancer and the knowledge required to understand the nature of the procedure is often one that cannot easily be bridged before the procedure needs to be performed.

If the procedures are performed while the child is awake, the younger child will typically need to be held down physically. The child therefore loses all sense of control and autonomy, and is entirely helpless. The parent must either collude in this or oppose it, but neither course relieves the child's sense that the familiar world, its boundaries and all of its supports are collapsing. As mentioned above, many of the procedures are performed on the patient's back, where he or she cannot see what is happening. This fear of the unknown is another powerful contributing factor in the experience of pain.

Finally, for older children there is often a sense of humiliation. Lumbar puncture and bone-marrow procedures require that part of the buttocks be exposed, not only to the doctor but to all the occupants of the room whom the child cannot see. This kind of helpless disruption of privacy can be profoundly distressing for some children.

In summary, interventions in paediatric oncology are often performed in an emotional and psychological environment that amplifies the physical experience of pain. It is hardly surprising, therefore, that the experience of invasive procedures is one which many children with cancer will remember with horror all of their lives.

There are four aspects of this multidimensional or holistic pain experience that can be addressed by a pharmacological approach. These are the physical discomfort, the awareness that the procedure is being performed, the fear caused by that knowledge, and finally the memory of the whole complex and traumatic experience.

Physical pain: need for analgesia

The physical experience of pain results from stimulation of sensory nerve endings in tissue that is damaged. The pain sensation travels as a series of electrical impulses through nerve fibres, via the spinal cord running through the spine, finally being recognised as pain in parts of the brain that are specialised for that function.

At all stages in its journey from the tissue to the brain, the sensation of pain is subject to modulation. This can be inhibitory, decreasing the pain or even abolishing it altogether (e.g. pain from sitting too long in one position is barely recognised consciously before the body acts on it by moving). It can also be amplified (e.g. after the initial trivial trauma, the pain of a wasp-sting increases as chemicals released in the sting stimulate and excite the nerve endings). Modulating factors can include other nerves that synapse with the pain fibres, or chemicals such as prostaglandins, cholecystokinin and substance P.

Even within the brain, the sense of pain can be altered. Intense pain can be manageable if it is understood and an end to it can be anticipated. On the other hand, pain that has no end may become intolerable even if the pain itself is mild. The pain of a wound acquired in battle may be easy to ignore until there is nothing else to take priority over it afterwards.

Thus capacity of the body to sense physical pain is sophisticated and dynamic, as its capacity to moderate the sensation of pain. Such a complex system offers a number of opportunities for therapeutic intervention using drugs.

Fear: need for anxiolysis

It has been seen that the fear and anxiety which attend painful procedures are unpleasant and require treatment in their own right. They also exacerbate the experience of pain, and management of anxiety is therefore an essential part of pain management. The major drugs used to treat anxiety are benzodiazepines (see below).

Superficially, a child who is drowsy may appear to be relaxed and not anxious. However, it is perfectly possible to induce drowsiness and by so doing to inhibit the expression of anxiety, while doing nothing at all to palliate the anxiety itself. For example, barbiturates and chloral hydrate are excellent sedatives but very poor anxiolytics.

Memory: need for amnestics

The memory of procedures performed during their illness remains with most children for the rest of their lives. Indeed, much of the long-term adverse impact of repeated interventions in paediatric oncology is associated with this cumulative experience, as one painful and frightening procedure succeeds another, each made worse by the memory of the last and the fear of the next one.

It may be considered that the importance of memory is such that the actual experience itself is of secondary significance. To base therapy on such an approach would be both cruel and deeply unethical. It is clearly unacceptable to allow a child to experience suffering simply on the grounds that we are able to intervene to abolish the memory of it. However, where a degree of suffering is unavoidable, drugs such as midazolam that can attenuate the memory of an unpleasant procedure have an important role. They must never be used alone in the management of painful procedures, as they are not analgesic and their anxiolytic effect is very short-lived.

Awareness: need for sleep

It is extremely difficult to perform many procedures on a child who is moving, so it is desirable both for the professional and for the patient that the child is as nearly unconscious as possible. Where deep sedation or general anaesthesia is unavailable or inappropriate, sedative medications are often used. These rarely allow a child to sleep through the procedure, but they can induce drowsiness. Again it is important not to confuse the drowsy child with one who is not anxious or distressed. For example, barbiturates or chloral hydrate will often help to make a child sleepy, and make it easier to perform procedures. However, they do very little to modify anxiety caused by the procedure.

Medications that can be helpful

Local anaesthetics

Perhaps the simplest local anaesthetic is ethyl chloride which, when sprayed on to a patch of skin, evaporates and in doing so activates superficial analgesic nerve pathways. These in turn inhibit the sensation of pain. The effect is small and short-lived.

More effective local anaesthetic agents (usually lidocaine or bupivacaine) are very useful for abolishing the experience of pain by simply 'switching off' the peripheral nerves that allow pain to be felt. Nerve cells usually function by transmitting electrical impulses. Different nerve fibres do this at different speeds depending on the nature of the fibre. For example, larger nerve fibres usually transmit impulses more quickly, as do those that are coated in a sheath of rapidly conducting myelin.

Ultimately, all information that is transmitted by nerve cells is a series of these electrical impulses. They are generated by means of charged ions, particularly potassium, sodium and chloride ions. Potassium ions are kept inside the cells, while sodium and chloride ions are kept outside them. This difference in concentrations is achieved through a series of pumps in the nerve-cell membrane which continually pump potassium ions into the cells and sodium and chloride ions out of them. As a result, there is a difference in electrical charge between the inside and the outside of the nerve-cell membrane. The pumps use a considerable amount of energy to maintain this situation. A sudden closing down of some of these pumps allows sodium to flow briefly but rapidly back into the cell, and it is this that constitutes the electrical impulse or action potential.

When there is no impulse travelling along it, the nerve-cell membrane is like a car in neutral on a downhill slope being held on the footbrake. Energy is required simply to prevent the car from going downhill. If the foot is relaxed, there is a surge of speed which can only be terminated by putting the foot back on the brake. This surge of speed is analogous to the action potential. A sequence of electrical impulses travels along a pain-sensitive nerve to the brain, where it is received as an experience of pain and interpreted in the sophisticated and complex manner described above.

Local anaesthetics reduce the magnitude, number and rate of spread of nerve impulses. To continue the car analogy, they put the handbrake on. They do this by blocking the channels in the nerve membrane through which sodium ions would normally travel, so that it is more difficult for an action potential to develop.

The practical upshot of this is that local anaesthetics work by a direct effect on the nerve-cell membrane itself. They will not work unless they are in contact with the nerve.

Topical anaesthetic creams such as EMLA (a eutectic mixture of lidocaine and prilocaine) or Ametop are absorbed through the skin and can anaesthetise the nerve endings immediately beneath them. The cream is spread over the patch of skin that needs to be anaesthetised and covered with a plastic covering. These measures are both safe and effective, but the cream needs to be left in place for at least 45 minutes. This can impose heavy restrictions in a busy children's outpatient clinic. However, many parents can learn to apply the cream before attending the clinic and its effectiveness and safety are such that for very minor procedures such as venepuncture this is probably the approach of choice.

To penetrate more deeply (e.g. to the bone marrow or other soft tissues), it is necessary to inject anaesthetic directly into the area concerned. The main difference between lidocaine and bupivacaine is their duration of action. The effects of bupivacaine can last for up to 45 minutes. No local anaesthetic agent provides long-lasting analgesia, although in other pain contexts local anaesthetics can be continuously infused to good effect.

General anaesthetics

Despite their widespread use and their very good safety profile in experienced hands, the mechanism by which general anaesthetics induce unconsciousness remains unclear. It seems likely that they act in a similar way to local anaesthetics in that they block sodium channels, perhaps by altering the nature of the membranes of nerve cells in the brain.

General anaesthetic agents may be given through a vein or inhaled as a gas through a mask. These alternatives make them very suitable for children, who will often express surprisingly sophisticated individual preferences.[10]

Common gaseous general anaesthetics include nitrous oxide, isoflurane, enflurane and halothane. These differ in the amount of the drug that needs to be inhaled before anaesthesia is achieved. Nitrous oxide is unusual among general anaesthetics in that it not only produces sleep, but is an extremely powerful analgesic. However, it is difficult to achieve general anaesthesia using this drug alone. Nitrous oxide, or laughing gas, has a very useful role at subanaesthetic doses in the management of pain associated with procedures. Mixed with oxygen in a 50%:50% mix, it is commercially available as Entonox (see below). This can be inhaled via a mask or mouthpiece immediately before or even during a painful procedure, and can provide very effective analgesia for those older children who are able to use it.

For paediatric patients who have central lines, induction of general anaesthesia by simply infusing the drug through the central line is a pain-free and anxiety-free experience. Intravenous anaesthetic agents include thiopentone and ketamine. Ketamine differs from thiopentone in that it is a very powerful analgesic. As an analgesic it acts in a somewhat unusual way, as it blocks some of the N-methyl D-aspartate (NMDA) pain receptors that are responsible for the physical memory of pain – that is, the receptors that make repeated painful procedures increasingly unpleasant. Ketamine is commonly used to obtain deep sedation but at lower doses, which are insufficient to put the patient to sleep, it is still a powerful sedative. However, it is structurally related to the recreational drug phenylcyclohexyl-piperidine (PCP), and at these doses it can produce hallucinations and unpleasant psychic experiences which mean it is poorly tolerated by many children. When used to achieve deep sedation and general anaesthesia in experienced hands it is a safe and effective drug.

Propofol is another intravenous anaesthetic that is commonly used to obtain general anaesthesia or deep sedation. In some respects it is ideal for paediatric oncology procedures, since it is associated with a rapid recovery, but this advantage may be offset by a small risk of convulsions some time after it has been used. Nevertheless, propofol is also a safe and effective drug.

Benzodiazepines

Benzodiazepine drugs such as diazepam (Valium) are both sedative and anxiolytic – that is, they not only encourage the child to fall asleep, but they also reduce the sensation of anxiety. They achieve this by interacting with receptors in the central nervous system, mostly in the cerebral cortex of the brain. There are at least two different types of receptor, and it has been suggested that it is through these types that benzodiazepines can exert their anti-anxiety effects on the one hand (Type 1) and their sedative effects on the other (Type 2). Although this is a convenient way to remember that the two functions are quite distinct, there is little experimental evidence to support this theory as an explanation for their mechanisms of action.

The ease with which benzodiazepines interact with their receptors is influenced by other neurotransmitters, in particular gamma-amino-butyric acid (GABA). It is believed that the receptors for GABA and benzodiazepines are closely linked, and that again the effect of both is to reduce the frequency with which the nerve fibres fire. As mentioned above, this may well be through channels in the nerve cell membranes, although it is likely that here chloride rather than sodium plays the major role.

Benzodiazepines are broken down in the liver, and many of the substances into which they are converted are themselves active and/or toxic, so the overall effect may be much longer-lived than that of the parent drug. As a class, benzodiazepines have lost much of their popularity since it became clear that many people who were prescribed them over a prolonged period found themselves unable easily to discontinue the drugs. This should not unduly influence the prescribing of benzodiazepines for children, as when they are used on an occasional basis, dependence does not occur. Furthermore, in children the drugs break down very quickly and are excreted promptly. This is in contrast to the situation in the elderly, for whom many of the drugs in this class were traditionally prescribed.

The relative effectiveness of benzodiazepines as anxiolytics and sedatives differs from one compound to another. The commonest benzodiazepines used to treat anxiety are diazepam (long half-life), lorazepam (intermediate half-life) and midazolam (short half-life). When selecting the most appropriate anxiolytic for management of an invasive procedure in children, the duration of action alone may not be the most important consideration. The benzodiazepines also differ in their capacity to induce amnesia,[11] and it is this action that makes the benzodiazepines such a valuable adjunct when preparing a child for an invasive procedure. Of the major benzodiazepines, lorazepam has some amnestic effect,[12] but it is midazolam that displays such an effect most consistently and effectively.[11,13–17] Midazolam can be administered as a nasal spray.[18]

Benzodiazepines have no analgesic activity and only a limited capacity to induce drowsiness in the context of acute discomfort. Taken alone they are not sufficient to prepare a child for a painful procedure.

Opioids

This very ancient class of drugs includes morphine and the other constituents of opium that have been used for thousands of years to alleviate insomnia and pain. Substances that are derived from morphine and other naturally occurring opioids are referred to as *opiates*, while the term *opioids* also includes synthetic or semi-synthetic derivatives (e.g. pethidine and fentanyl).

Opioids act by mimicking the effect of molecules produced naturally by the body. They act on receptors in the brain and induce powerful analgesia. They also act on other centres in the brain and elsewhere to produce side-effects such as nausea and vomiting, reduced respiratory rate, and constipation.

For convenience, in this section we shall consider morphine first, and then the other opioids only in so far as they differ from it.

Morphine can be taken by mouth, intravenously or subcutaneously. The intramuscular route is usually contraindicated in children, as any theoretical advantage in drug delivery is more than offset by the discomfort of the injection. Once absorbed, morphine is converted in the liver to a number of different substances, some of which are inactive, while others are more potent than morphine itself. Morphine acts on receptors in the brain and must therefore pass from the blood into the brain tissue. It appears to do this very effectively in children, as in adults, and is then excreted via the kidneys.

Morphine is a very powerful analgesic. It also has an impact on mood, often lifting it (euphoria). It can also induce feelings of strangeness or even sadness (dysphoria). In adults, morphine can induce nausea and vomiting, although this side-effect appears to be relatively unusual in children. Children do become easily constipated by morphine, and there is a risk of urinary retention in childhood that seems to exceed that in adulthood. Most of these are problems associated with multiple dosing of morphine rather than the single dose which is administered in preparation for an invasive procedure. There is also a risk of a decrease in respiratory rate and blood pressure. These adverse effects are usually counteracted by the experience of pain, but if too much morphine is administered before a painful procedure, there is no such counteracting stimulus and apnoea may very rarely result.

It is often assumed that children are more sensitive than adults to the adverse effects of morphine. This is probably true in children under one year old. However, older children appear if anything to be rather resistant to the effects of morphine, and to require higher doses per unit weight than their adult counterparts. This is probably related to the rate at which they are able to excrete morphine.[19–30]

The latter half of the twentieth century saw an increase in concern about addiction associated with the use of morphine that is quite out of proportion to the real risks. Such concern should not deter clinicians from using morphine in a therapeutic setting, where the risk of addiction is extremely low.

Synthetic opioids that have been developed more recently include fentanyl, which is very much more powerful than morphine, and may have a slightly better adverse effects profile, particularly in children.[31] It is not available by mouth, but has been successfully administered in a lollipop formulation.[32]

Diamorphine, another naturally occurring opioid, is slightly more powerful than morphine and has the advantage of being highly soluble, so higher doses can be given without increasing the volume of an injection. In other respects it is otherwise very similar to morphine.

Given the excellent safety profile of these opioids, it is unclear why many paediatric oncology centres choose instead to use pethidine. Pethidine is a relatively weak opioid which is broken down by the body into toxic metabolites that accumulate in the brain and can induce convulsions. The incidence of dysphoria is very high. Nevertheless, pethidine has enjoyed a great vogue in North America.[16,33,34]

Generally speaking, the role of opioids in procedures associated with paediatric oncology should probably be limited to administration during general anaesthetic or deep sedation for bone-marrow procedures where the level of pain is intense. Once again, however, they are not sufficient on their own, as although morphine and other opioids are excellent analgesics, they are indifferent sedatives and do not influence anxiety.

Others

Chloral hydrate

There is a long tradition in paediatrics of the use of chloral hydrate for the management of very minor procedures. The drug is administered orally but does not always have a pleasant taste, and it can provoke nausea in some children. Furthermore, the concentration is such that for larger children the volume they are required to take may simply be intolerable. Some North American literature suggests that it can be given rectally,[33] but this is not common practice in the UK.

Chloral is usually considered to be a very safe drug, although this may simply be because very little of it is typically taken in by the child. It has very few adverse effects on the central nervous system or cardiovascular system. However, children with renal impairment become more sensitive to side-effects, and chloral can also enhance the effects of other medications on these systems. Chloral is activated in the liver by hepatic alcohol dehydrogenase to form an active compound (trichloroethanol). Prescribing it for patients with liver failure is therefore both ineffective and potentially dangerous, as it may precipitate coma.

Chloral hydrate has no anxiolytic or analgesic properties. These limitations, combined with the difficulty that many children have in tolerating it, mean that it has little role in the modern management of paediatric oncology procedures.

Barbiturates

Barbiturates act directly on the central nervous system to induce sedation. They are not commonly used in the UK, but have in the past been popular in the USA.[33] This was largely because of the rapid onset and offset of the drug's effects.[35] Although an overdose of barbiturates can induce apnoea, aspiration and severe cardiovascular depression,[36] in sedative doses the risk of these effects is very small.

It is now known that the effect of barbiturates on pain perception may in fact be to increase sensitivity to painful procedures.[33] They should now probably be regarded as contraindicated for children undergoing invasive procedures. Barbiturates are not anxiolytic and do not induce amnesia.

Entonox

Nitrous oxide is a gas that is capable of providing very good analgesia without the need for oral or parenteral administration. It is usually administered as Entonox, a 50% mixture with oxygen.[37] The incidence of dysphoria seems to be rather low, and much more commonly patients experience an elevation of mood. For this reason it is known as 'laughing gas'. It appears to be very safe,[38] but in high concentrations it may induce loss of consciousness and therefore pose the risk of aspiration of the contents of the stomach into the lungs. These are probably small risks, but the use of Entonox has not been well researched in children and, as with other techniques for managing the pain of invasive procedures, it has probably now been superseded by the development of newer anaesthetic and deep sedation techniques.

Cannabinoids

In adolescents, derivatives of marijuana such as nabilone can have a significant impact on the manifestations of anticipatory anxiety. These include nausea and vomiting, but such anxiety can also exacerbate the multidimensional experience of pain.

Phenothiazines

This class of drugs includes promethazine (Phenergan). Phenothiazines are remarkable for the diversity of their useful effects, which include sedation, a decrease in respiratory secretions and anti-emesis, but not anxiolysis, amnesia or analgesia. They are not commonly used in the UK.

Using medication to help children who are undergoing procedures

It has already been suggested that it is important to distinguish between the different therapeutic effects that can be achieved by using drugs. Drugs that are effective anxiolytics may be indifferent or quite ineffective analgesics. Most pharmacological approaches therefore utilise a combination of medications designed to address different aspects of the pain experience.

Broadly speaking, there are two groups of approaches. First, there are approaches that render the child unconscious (general anaesthesia or deep sedation). Unconsciousness on its own does not guarantee analgesia, and such an approach should be combined with some form of analgesia. Secondly, there is a much wider range of pharmacological combinations that leave the child conscious during procedures (for the purposes of this chapter, this group of approaches is described as conscious sedation).

Conscious sedation

General anaesthesia and deep sedation are highly effective and incur little risk to the patient. Performing invasive procedures on a conscious child should be the exception rather than the rule. However, there are some situations in which it is unavoidable. Financial considerations may make access to anaesthetists difficult, and some older children may prefer to avoid a general anaesthetic.

The ideal intervention for management of painful procedures would offer sedation, anxiolysis, amnesia and analgesia. No single medication can offer all of these. Therefore one solution to the problem is to combine drugs with different characteristics, in an attempt to achieve all four aims.

The most widely used combination is that of an opioid and an anxiolytic.[33,34,39] In the past, a combination of pethidine and lorazepam or diazepam was favoured. Midazolam is now becoming increasingly popular,[11,13–15,17,18,40–49] and has been combined with morphine, fentanyl or ketamine.[16]

The popularity of conscious sedation may be explained in part by the perceived advantage to the physician or nurse in having a child who is conscious throughout the procedure. A definition of conscious sedation by the American Academy of Pediatrics[50] suggests that, in addition to maintaining protective reflexes and an airway, a patient should be able to respond to physical stimulation or verbal commands. For most invasive procedures, a child who is able to respond in this way should probably no longer be considered to be adequately sedated. On the other hand, conscious sedation would clearly be inappropriately toxic for much more minor procedures, such as venepuncture.

Thus the risk is that most drug combinations are too toxic for minor procedures, and provide inadequate preparation for more major ones. It is difficult to see the place of conscious sedation in modern management of procedure-related pain in children, and indeed it is rarely used in the UK. A move away from performing procedures on conscious children has long been anticipated in the USA,[33] but is happening only very slowly.

Deep sedation and general anaesthesia

Deep sedation is distinguished from general anaesthesia by the fact that the patient, although unconscious, is able to maintain his or her airway and therefore does not require intubation. Nevertheless, it should only be performed by an anaesthetist with anaesthetic equipment readily available. The drugs employed are usually propofol and ketamine. Both are injected intravenously, usually through a central venous line.

It is perfectly possible for an unconscious patient to experience and respond physiologically to pain. Ketamine, but not propofol, has an analgesic as well as anaesthetic action. Both drugs are very effective in children. The risk of respiratory depression is extremely small, and in the presence of an anaesthetist with appropriate equipment it presents little danger to the patient.

Bone-marrow aspirations and trephines are extremely painful, and an opioid, usually morphine or fentanyl, should be given even to the unconscious patient if these procedures are to be performed. In addition, many oncologists infiltrate the area with local anaesthetic such as lidocaine. The skin, periosteum and even the marrow itself can be infiltrated.

Lidocaine may be effective for up to half an hour, but the effects of marcaine last much longer. If a lumbar puncture is the only procedure to be performed under the anaesthetic, opioids are probably unnecessary.

The benefit of deep sedation is that it is safe and highly effective both in abolishing pain and in minimising cumulative anxiety and distress during repeated procedures. However, children who are to have deep sedation must fast for several hours before the procedure, and this can be a source of some discomfort.

A general anaesthetic has all the advantages of deep sedation, but is a more major undertaking, requiring intubation and artificial ventilation. General anaesthesia is able to provide a very stable haemodynamic and respiratory environment during the procedure and is therefore very appropriate for longer procedures.

General anaesthesia can be induced using intravenous or inhalational agents. The use of frequent, repeated anaesthetics employing either method is very safe in children.[2–4,51]

Once again, anaesthesia alone is not sufficient to secure analgesia, and these agents will usually be combined with opioids and/or local anaesthetic infiltration at the site. Recovery following a very short general anaesthetic, such as that required for lumbar puncture or a bone-marrow procedure, is extremely rapid. Such cases can be managed as day-case procedures with no ill effects. However, like deep sedation, a general anaesthetic requires the child to be fasted for several hours. Failure to comply can result in the need to delay procedures and therefore, on occasion, chemotherapy.

Procedures in the conscious patient: weighing up cost and benefit

It is no longer necessary for a child to experience pain during an invasive procedure in the management of cancer. For very minor procedures we now have effective topical local anaesthetic creams that do not even need to be injected to provide numbness and very good analgesia. Most children who are undergoing treatment for cancer have surgically implanted devices that allow blood to be taken and chemotherapy to be administered with a minimum of needle-pricks, and sometimes without the need for needles at all. For more major procedures there is a range of techniques that render the child rapidly unconscious so that the procedure can be performed with the minimum of trauma, and then allow the child to be swiftly woken up and ready to go home well on the same day. Why then do children still have to experience such pain?

There is a clear reluctance in some centres to offer adequate sedation to children to ensure that they are not conscious during traumatic procedures. Performing invasive procedures on conscious children appears to be culturally much more acceptable in North America than in the UK.[8]

This is probably due to differences in both medical and popular culture, and especially concern about the risk of litigation. There is a tendency for professionals working in a litigious social climate to consider it far worse to do something potentially dangerous than to fail to do something beneficial. In the context of this cautious medical approach, the burden of evidence may have to be very heavily in favour of safety before a procedure is embraced by the medical establishment. In other words, repeated general anaesthetic may be seen to be 'guilty until proven innocent'. In fact, there is abundant evidence to suggest that repeated deep sedation and general anaesthetic are perfectly safe. Unfortunately, once it is believed that a procedure is dangerous, it can be difficult to become convinced otherwise.

Finally, in a private healthcare system, expense can be a major consideration when dictating a clinical approach. The administration of deep sedation or anaesthetic requires trained personnel to be available as well as specialised equipment and a clinical area in which the procedure can safely take place. The extra expense incurred by this approach becomes very considerable. Furthermore, the need to involve an anaesthetist imposes logistical complications[52] that must be taken into consideration if 'time is money'.

Against these very real concerns must be set the need to protect the child from pain and trauma, which for many procedures can be achieved at best only incompletely if the child remains conscious. As evidence accumulates to suggest that pain in childhood, particularly if repeated, can have long-term adverse effects,[5–7] it may be that there will be a growing tendency for inadequately managed suffering itself to become the grounds for legal action. Perhaps litigation will succeed where scientific evidence has failed in encouraging paediatric oncology centres to offer anaesthesia rather than conscious sedation.

Summary and conclusion

In the past, the experience of children with cancer was one of recurrent and unending anguish as – with each successive procedure – fear, anxiety and pain became worse. This pain occurred in a context that included the terror of separation, the possibility of death and loss, unpleasant physical sensations such as nausea and vomiting, and a changing self-image as steroids made children fat, and chemotherapy made their hair fall out.

We are not yet in a position to influence some of these problems. However, we are able to moderate or even abolish completely the quartet of anxiety, awareness, unpleasant memory and – perhaps above all – pain. If we are to change a culture that has traditionally regarded suffering in children as acceptable and sometimes even necessary in the child's best interests, we must continue to record and report the safety and effectiveness of approaches that can avoid completely the pain of procedures in childhood cancer.

References

1 McGraw M (1941) Neural maturation as exemplified in the changing reactions of the infant to pin prick. *Child Dev.* **12**: 31–42.

2 McDowall RH, Scher CS and Barst SM (1995) Total intravenous anesthesia for children undergoing brief diagnostic or therapeutic procedures. *J Clin Anesth.* **7**: 273–80.

3 Scheiber G, Ribeiro FC, Karpienski H and Strehl K (1996) Deep sedation with propofol in preschool children undergoing radiation therapy. *Paediatr Anaesth.* **6**: 209–13.

4 Hain WR, Tomlinson JH and Barbor PRH (1985) Anaesthesia for minor procedures in children with malignant disease. *J R Soc Med.* **78**: 715–20.

5   Taddio A, Goldbach M, Ipp M, Stevens B and Koren G (1995) Effect of neonatal circumcision on pain responses during vaccination in boys. *Lancet.* **345**: 291–2.

6   Fitzgerald M, Millard C and MacIntosh N (1988) Hyperalgesia in premature infants. *Lancet.* **1**: 292.

7   Anand KJS (1997) Long-term effects of pain in neonates and infants. In: TS Jensen, JA Turner and Z Wiesenfeld-Hallin (eds) *Proceedings of the Eighth World Congress on Pain, 1997 Vancouver.* IASP Press, Seattle, WA, 881–92.

8   Hain RDW and Campbell C (2001) Invasive procedures carried out in conscious chidren: contrast between North American and European paediatric oncology centres. *Arch Dis Child.* **85**: 12–15.

9   Bertoni F, Bonardi A, Magno L *et al.* (1999) Hypnosis instead of general anaesthesia in paediatric radiotherapy: report of three cases. *Radiother Oncol.* **52**: 185–90.

10 Tierney E, Ritchie PA, Hain WR and Cooke RA (1985) Halothane or enflurane for inhalation induction? A study of children's preferences. *Anesth Analg.* **64**: 77–9.

11 Veselis RA, Reinsel RA, Feshchenko VA and Wronski M (1997) The comparative amnestic effects of midazolam, propofol, thiopental and fentanyl at equisedative concentrations. *Anesthesiology.* **87**: 749–64.

12 Henry DW, Burwinkle JW and Klutman NE (1991) Determination of sedative and amnestic doses of lorazepam in children. *Clin Pharm.* **10**: 625–9.

13 Wagner BK, O'Hara DA and Hammond JS (1997) Drugs for amnesia in the ICU. *Am J Crit Care.* **6**: 192–201.

14 Shields RE (1997) A comprehensive review of sedative and analgesic agents. *Crit Care Nurs Clin North Am.* **9**: 281–8.

15 Sectish TC (1997) Use of sedation and local anesthesia to prepare children for procedures. *Am Fam Physician.* **55**(3): 909–16.

16 Marx CM, Stein J, Tyler MK, Nieder ML, Shurin SB and Blumer JL (1997) Ketamine–midazolam versus meperidine–midazolam for painful procedures in pediatric oncology patients. *J Clin Oncol.* **15**: 94–102.

17 Craney JM and Gorman LN (1997) Conscious sedation and implantable devices. Safe and effective sedation during pacemaker and implantable cardioverter defibrillator placement. *Crit Care Nurs Clin North Am.* **9**: 325–34.

18 Ljungman G, Kreuger A, Andreasson S, Gordh T and Sorensen S (2000) Midazolam nasal spray reduces procedural anxiety in children. *Pediatrics.* **105**: 73–8.

19 Hain RDW, Hardcastle A, Pinkerton CR and Aherne GW (1999) Morphine and morphine-6-glucuronide in the plasma and cerebrospinal fluid of children. *Br J Clin Pharmacol.* **48**: 37–42.

20 Choonara IA, McKay P, Hain R and Rane A (1989) Morphine metabolism in children. *Br J Clin Pharmacol.* **28**: 599–604.

21 Dagan O, Klein J, Bohn D, Barker G and Koren G (1993) Morphine pharmacokinetics in children following cardiac surgery: effects of disease and inotropic support. *J Cardiothor Vasc Anesth.* **7**: 396–8.

22 Dahlström B, Bolme P, Feychting H, Noack G and Paalzow L (1979) Morphine pharmacokinetics in children. *Clin Pharmacol Ther.* **26**: 354–65.

23 Chinyanga HM, Vandenberge H, Bohn D, Macleod S and Soldin S (1983) Pharmacokinetics of morphine in young children following cardiac surgery. *Anesthesiology.* **59**: A447.

24 McRorie TI, Lynn AM, Nespeca MK, Opheim KE and Slattery JT (1992) The maturation of morphine clearance and metabolism. *Am J Dis Child.* **146**: 972–6.

25 Mickell JJ, Pedigo A, Lucking SE and Albert MA (1990) Age-related differences in the use of morphine, diazepam and pancuronium for mechanically ventilated children. *Dev Pharmacol Ther.* **14**: 20–8.

26 Nahata MC, Miser AW, Reuning RH (1985) Variation in morphine pharmacokinetics in children with cancer. *Dev Pharmacol Ther.* **8**: 182–8.

27 Hunt AM, Joel S, Dick G and Goldman A (1999) Population pharmacokinetics of oral morphine and its glucuronides in children receiving morphine as immediate release liquid or sustained-release tablets for cancer pain. *J Pediatrics.* **135**(1): 47–55.

28 Olkkola KT, Maunskela E-L, Korpela R and Rosenberg PH (1988) Kinetics and dynamics of postoperative intravenous morphine in children. *Clin Pharmacol Ther.* **44**: 128–36.

29 Shelly MP, Cory EP and Park GR (1986) Pharmacokinetics of morphine in two children before and after liver transplantation. *Br J Anaesth.* **58**: 1218–23.

30 Vanderberghe H, MacLeod S, Chinyanga M, Endrenyi L and Soldin S (1983) Pharmacokinetics of intravenous morphine in balanced anesthesia: studies on children. *Drug Metab Rev.* **14**: 887–903.

31 Hertzka RE, Fisher DM, Gauntlett IS and Spellman BS (1987) Are infants sensitive to respiratory depression from fentanyl? *Anesthesiology.* **67**: A512.

32 Schechter NL, Weisman SJ, Rosenblum M, Bernstein B and Conard PL (1995) The use of oral transmucosal fentanyl citrate for painful procedures in children. *Pediatrics.* **95**: 335–9.

33 Zeltzer LK, Jay SM and Fisher DM (1989) The management of pain associated with pediatric procedures. *Pediatr Clin North Am.* **36**: 941–64.

34 Cook BA, Bass JW, Nomizu S and Alexander ME (1992) Sedation of children for technical procedures: current standard of practice. *Clin Pediatr.* **31**: 137–42.

35 Varner PD, Ebert JP, McKay RD (1985) Methohexital sedation of children undergoing CT scan. *Anesth Analg.* **64**: 643–5.

36 Harvey SC (1985) Hypnotics and sedatives. In: AG Gilman, LS Goodman, TW Rall and F Murad (eds) *The Pharmacological Basis of Therapeutics* (7e). Macmillan Publishing Company, New York, 339–71.

37 Warren VN, Crawford AN and Young TM (1983) The use of Entonox as a sedation agent for children who have refused operative dentistry. *J Dent.* **11**: 306–12.

38 Griffin GC, Campbell VD and Jones R (1981) Nitrous oxide–oxygen sedation for minor surgery. *J Am Acad Pediatr.* **245**: 2411–13.

39 Pohlgeers AP, Friedland LR and Keegan JL (1995) Combination fentanyl and diazepam for pediatric conscious sedation. *Acad Emerg Med.* **2**: 879–83.

40 Broennle AM and Cohen DE (1993) Pediatric anesthesia and sedation. *Curr Opin Pediatr.* **5**: 310–4.

41 Ly IC and Tan CL (1992) Use of intravenous midazolam for sedation in children undergoing ward procedures. *J Sing Paediatr Soc.* **34**: 30–3.

42 Kupietzky A and Houpt MI (1993) Midazolam: a review of its use for conscious sedation of children. *Pediatr Dent.* **15**: 237–41.

43 Lewis JH and Benjamin SB (1990) Safety of midazolam and diazepam for conscious sedation. *J Clin Gastroenterol.* **12**: 716–7.

44 Nordt SP and Clark RF (1997) Midazolam: a review of therapeutic uses and toxicity. *J Emerg Med.* **15**: 357–65.

45 Rosen DA and Rosen KR (1998) Intravenous conscious sedation with midazolam in paediatric patients. *Int J Clin Pract.* **52**: 46–50.

46 Sandler ES, Weyman C and Conner K (1992) Midazolam versus fentanyl as premedication for painful procedures in children with cancer. *Pediatrics.* **89**: 631–4.

47 Sievers TD, Yee JD, Foley ME, Blanding PJ and Berde CB (1991) Midazolam for conscious sedation during pediatric oncology procedures: safety and recovery parameters. *Pediatrics.* **88**: 1172–9.

48 Wright SW, Chudnofsky CR, Dronen SC *et al.* (1993) Comparison of midazolam and diazepam for conscious sedation in the emergency department. *Ann Emerg Med.* **22**: 201–5.

49 Yaster M, Nichols DG and Deshpande J (1990) Midazolam–fentanyl intravenous sedation in children: case report of respiratory arrest. *Pediatrics.* **86**: 463–7.

50 American Academy of Pediatrics Committee on Drugs (1992) Guidelines for the monitoring and management of pediatric patients during and after sedation for diagnostic and therapeutic procedures. *Pediatrics.* **89**: 1110–16.

51 Wark H, O'Halloran M and Overton J (1986) Prospective study of liver function in children following multiple anaesthetics at short intervals. *Br J Anaesth.* **58**(11): 1224–8.

52 Bubien RS, Fisher JD, Gentzel JA *et al.* (1998) North American Society of Pacing and Electrophysiology (NASPE) expert consensus document: use of iv (conscious) sedation/analgesia by non-anesthesia personnel in patients undergoing arrhythmia-specific diagnostic, therapeutic and surgical procedures. *Pacing Clin Electrophysiol.* **21**: 375–85.

4

The psychological management of paediatric procedure-related cancer pain. Part 1

Christina Liossi

Introduction

Many methods are cited in the literature for managing paediatric pain, and they are commonly grouped under the headings *pharmacological* and *non-pharmacological or psychological* methods. Although pharmacological methods are quite effective, their use in the clinical setting is still hindered by a number of misconceptions as well as lack of knowledge regarding their longer-term safety in the treatment of pain in children. Children's distress and coping behaviours during acute painful medical procedures are important areas of study in paediatric psychology. Various psychological intervention techniques, such as distraction, imagery, relaxation, cognitive therapy and hypnosis, have effectively promoted coping and decreased children's acute and chronic pain in recent years.

This chapter focuses on the psychological management of procedure-related cancer pain. The first part describes and evaluates interventions such as preparation, deep breathing, distraction, play therapy, relaxation and cognitive therapy, while the second part discusses exclusively clinical hypnosis. Special emphasis is placed on cognitive therapy and hypnosis because they have achieved status as *empirically validated* interventions in paediatric procedure-related pain management. For all of the interventions presented here, first the fundamental principles underlying their use are discussed, then the representative research studies that have evaluated the approach are reviewed, and finally each section concludes with a description of the techniques that are widely used in actual clinical practice.

Management of procedure-related pain in paediatric oncology

The goals of pain management for paediatric procedures are to minimise the patient's suffering and facilitate a successful procedure. The management of pain associated with paediatric procedures is not a simple task. There are multiple approaches to and philosophies regarding the treatment of procedure-related pain. Different treatment approaches are practised both at different treatment centres in different countries, and by individual practitioners within the same setting. One extreme is the practice of providing no pharmacological support and no or only limited psychological support, based on the belief that the pain is time limited, the risk of medication is unwarranted, and the procedure is being performed for the child's benefit. Under these circumstances, children often need to be restrained by several nurses.

At the other extreme is the administration of pharmacological interventions without any psychological support, based on the belief that the pain is very intense, that pharmacological agents facilitate the procedure medically, and that they are sufficient to address the pain and distress associated with the procedure. There are many alternatives to these extremes (*see* Figure 4.1), and the ideal approach is a judicious combination of pharmacological and psychological approaches depending on the specific procedure and the individual child.

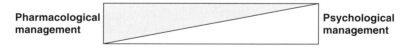

Figure 4.1:   Treatment approaches to paediatric procedure-related cancer pain.

Psychological management of paediatric procedure-related cancer pain

The aims of psychological interventions when used alone or in combination with pharmacological treatments in the management of procedure-related pain are as follows:

- to decrease the patient's pain, anxiety and general distress before, during and after the procedure
- to promote active coping with pain and cancer in general
- to assist patients in reconceptualising their view of themselves from being passive, reactive and helpless to being active, resourceful and competent
- to prevent the development of dysfunctional and maladaptive schemata.[4.1]

Psychological interventions for acute pain associated with medical procedures are more likely to be successful if certain principles are followed. These include the following:

- organising and presenting information in conceptual categories in both verbal and written form
- presenting information gradually, to avoid overwhelming the patient
- individualising interventions
- assessing the patient's understanding by asking them to describe what they will do before, during and after a medical procedure
- including the patient's family in the treatment programme.

The psychological interventions most commonly used in clinical practice (*see* Figure 4.2) and significant issues related to their use are discussed below, after a brief consideration of the importance of the treatment room and developmental issues that are pertinent to the use of psychological interventions.

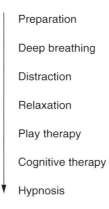

Preparation

Deep breathing

Distraction

Relaxation

Play therapy

Cognitive therapy

Hypnosis

Figure 4.2:   Psychological analgesic interventions in order of increasing complexity.

4.1   A schema is a relatively enduring unit of belief from which moment-to-moment cognitions are derived. These schemata are the rules that govern how an individual assigns meaning. They form the basis of the consistency of interpretations of a particular set of situations by an individual.

The treatment room

The environment in which procedures are administered must be comfortable and non-threatening. In virtually every circumstance, the child's bed and room should not be the location for a painful procedure. Every attempt should be made to eliminate environmental stresses, such as loud noises, cold tables and discharging beepers, because they increase the child's distress. In addition, in many tertiary-care medical centres, the least experienced person is assigned the task of performing a painful procedure. Every effort should be made to ensure that the person who performs the procedure has proficient technical skills.

Developmental considerations relating to the use of psychological interventions with children

When working with children, the healthcare professional is continually confronted with the challenge of determining the most effective therapeutic strategy, based on medical and psychological needs as well as developmental level.[4.2] Psychological interventions are in part a medium by which patients are allowed to transform cognitive or language-coded information into a physical or emotional response. Thus if interventions are to be effective, they must be made at the level at which the patient has processing competency.

Preparation

Fundamental principles

Preparation is the commonest psychological intervention for children who undergo medical procedures. It is a generic term for a number of techniques and procedures, the central component of which is provision of information to the child and their parents concerning the necessity, nature and various phases of the impending medical procedure. The rationale underlying preparatory interventions is that unexpected stress

4.2   A broad range of physical, cognitive, linguistic, emotional and social stages.

is more anxiety provoking and more difficult to cope with than anticipated or predictable stress.[1] Children who undergo systematic preparation, rehearsal and supportive care respond best before, during and after the procedure. Therefore adequate information and communication with the patient are of vital importance.

Preparatory information can be characterised as being sensory or procedural.[2] Procedural information involves the depiction of the steps of the procedure, without descriptions of sensations. Sensory information involves a description of the sensations that the patient will experience at various points in the procedure. For example, a child who is being prepared for a lumbar puncture might be told that the cleansing of their back will feel 'cold', whereas the numbing medicine will feel like a 'pinch' or a 'prick'. The type of information that is most effective appears to be a combination of sensory and procedural data.[3] Although widely used in clinical practice, the efficacy of this intervention has not been evaluated in research.

Specific techniques used

In actual clinical practice, preparation involves the following components:

- introducing the child to medical personnel
- giving the child developmentally appropriate information about what will be done and how it will feel
- letting the child handle equipment
- having the child practise the procedure on a doll
- discussion of the child's feelings and thoughts about the procedure.

Various methods have been used to provide children with information about medical procedures (painful or not), including doll play, hospital tours, story and colouring books, and cognitive strategies.[4]

Despite wide agreement about the benefits of preparing children for procedures, there have been few attempts in the literature to establish clear guidelines about how young patients should be prepared for their treatments. There are three phases involved in performing a medical procedure where adequate preparation is relevant. These phases, and a summary of the key steps within each of them, are presented next and are also shown schematically in Figure 4.3.

Phase One involves preparation before the procedure, and consists of explaining to the patient in clear, developmentally appropriate language why the procedure is needed, what will happen and how it will feel. The

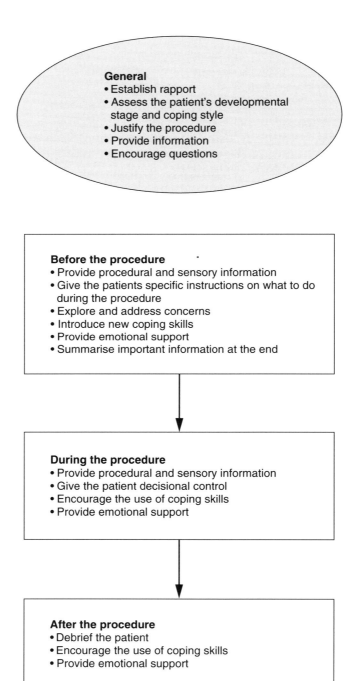

Figure 4.3:   Steps involved in adequate preparation for a medical procedure.[5]

patient must be given the opportunity to ask questions and express concerns. An assessment of the patient's coping style can be conducted in order to suggest appropriate coping strategies.

Phase Two involves care during the procedure. During the procedure the health professionals can, if the patient wants this and is conscious, explain what is going on and how it is likely to feel, and encourage and reinforce the patient's attempts to practise coping strategies. It is important that children are given decisional control over the procedure, rather than absolute or behavioural control. With decisional control, the child may be offered, for example, the choice of the procedure beginning in three or seven seconds rather than after an indefinite delay, as is typical of behavioural control. Giving children limitless control leaves them to their own devices with regard to how to manage themselves in the situation, and increases their anxiety.

Finally, *Phase Three* involves care during the recovery phase. During this phase it is useful to debrief the young patient and encourage them to take an active part in recovery efforts. The patient can continue to use their coping skills.

Further research and controlled clinical trials will be necessary to evaluate which of these steps will be most helpful to individual patients. However, as each patient suffers in their own unique way, clinical sensitivity must always take priority over general guidelines.

Time optimisation for preparation

The optimum time for preparation for medical procedures is crucial. Too little time for preparation is associated with higher levels of distress and anxiety, but too much time can result in increased anticipatory anxiety. Figure 4.4 demonstrates the relationship between anxiety and time prior to the procedure when the preparation is given. The optimum time for preparation is individual specific.

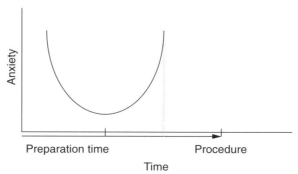

Figure 4.4:   Time of preparation vs. experienced anxiety.

Deep breathing

Deep breathing quickly sends a signal to the entire body to relax. There are no reports available on the usefulness of deep breathing in isolation from other strategies for procedure-related pain control, although it is a component of many relaxation procedures that have been researched. Deep breathing is the most easily learned of the relaxation techniques, and very little training is needed in order to obtain benefits. For patients in intense acute pain or undergoing a stressful but not painful procedure, deep breathing may be the most that they can achieve. It can also be quite effective in capturing and holding a very distressed patient's attention, and may be the first step towards using imagery to distract the patient further from the distress of the moment.

Whenever the young patient, especially during invasive procedures, notices some tension in their body, or they feel fearful or anxious, they can practise deep breathing by following several simple steps.

1   Make your position as comfortable as you can wherever you are.
2   Now begin to focus on your breathing. Pay attention to how it feels to breathe in and out, breathing in easily and deeply, holding your breath for a moment and then exhaling fully.
3   Inhale deeply through your nose while counting slowly to 5. (To assist the young child in doing this you can ask them to imagine that they are a big tyre or a colourful balloon being inflated. A picture of Michelin's tyre man or pictures of balloons can assist this imagery (*see* Figure 4.5).
4   As you inhale, pull the air into your abdomen, then through your entire chest and upward to your shoulders. Notice your chest moving up and your shoulders moving back as you breathe in deeply.
5   Hold your breath for a few moments.
6   Exhale through your mouth, making a relaxing, whooshing sound like the wind as you blow out to a slow count of 5. (The younger patient can imagine blowing out a candle really carefully, or blowing an imaginary feather off their nose or their mother's nose.)
7   As you exhale, let your breath go from the bottom of your abdomen up through your chest and all the way up to your shoulders. Notice your chest moving down and your shoulders moving forward as you breathe out all of the air.
8   Continue breathing deeply for several minutes.
9   When you have learned to relax yourself using deep breathing, practise this whenever and wherever you feel yourself getting tense.

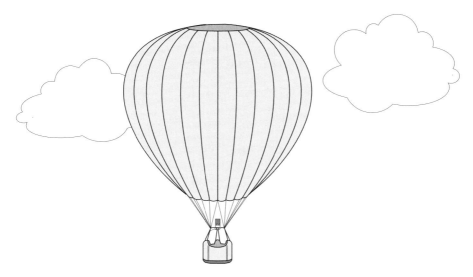

Figure 4.5:   Pictures can assist deep breathing.

An alternative form of this technique includes blowing bubbles (e.g. 'Imagine you are blowing bubbles. Blow some really big ones. Now blow some small ones. Continue blowing for several minutes').

Distraction

Fundamental principles

Distraction or attentional diversion can be an excellent coping strategy for patients who are in pain or distress. The pain is not going to increase and the consequences are not going to be detrimental if they do not remain constantly preoccupied with the stressful situation in which they are. Distraction involves helping the patient to learn to refocus attention away from the stressor (e.g. pain) and on to something else. This strategy can encompass a wide range of distractions that are incompatible with the experience of severe pain. Patients can be taught to divert their attention externally or internally in fantasy. External diversions include studying one's surroundings and concentrating or meditating on some external focus point. Internal or fantasy diversion includes mentally going to one's favourite place, or to any place where one feels comfortable and safe, and remembering what it feels like to perform a pleasant activity. In addition, a patient might fantasise about transforming the contextual circumstances into something dramatic, such as being their favourite undercover operative or detective hero who is recovering from a bullet wound.

Efficacy in clinical pain

Distraction techniques are often effective and are easily implemented. A number of simple, distraction-type interventions, such as distraction by music via headphones,[6] nurse-implemented distraction,[7] and a variety of relatively simple distraction techniques implemented by parents,[8–10] have been empirically evaluated and shown to be effective in reducing pain and distress associated with paediatric procedures.

Cohen and colleagues[11] evaluated a low-cost and practical intervention designed to decrease the distress of children, parents and nurses during children's immunisations. The intervention consisted of distraction in the form of children viewing a popular cartoon movie and being coached by nurses and parents to attend to the movie. Nurses' coaching consisted of comments about the movie (e.g. 'Tell me what is happening in the movie'), as well as direct suggestions ('Watch the movie'). Specific times for prompting the children included procedural junctures (e.g. prior to cleaning the site or prior to the injection) whenever the child was attending to the nurse activities, and whenever the child appeared to be distressed. A total of 92 children, aged 4–6 years, and their parents were alternatively assigned to a nurse coach intervention, a nurse coach plus training parent and child intervention, or a standard medical care condition. The results indicated that, in the two-intervention conditions, children coped better and were less distressed, nurses and parents exhibited more coping-promoting behaviour, and parents and nurses were less distressed than in the control condition. Although neither intervention was superior with regard to any of the variables assessed in the study, the nurse coach intervention was markedly more practical and cost-effective.

Vessey and colleagues[12] investigated the effectiveness of a distraction technique in reducing a child's perceived pain and behavioural distress during venepunctures. A total of 100 children (aged 3–12 years) scheduled for routine blood sampling were recruited and randomly assigned to an experimental or control group. During venepuncture, the control subjects received standard preparation, which consisted of being comforted by means of physical touch and soft voices, while the experimental subjects were encouraged to use a kaleidoscope as a distraction technique. The results indicated that the experimental group perceived less pain and displayed less behavioural distress than the control group.

Mason and colleagues[13] assessed the effectiveness of two simple distraction procedures for reducing children's pain and distress during accessing of implanted drug delivery systems (Port-A-Caths) and external semi-permanent catheters (Hickman lines). Three conditions (control, brief film and short story) were delivered during repeated medical procedures in a randomised sequence to eight young children with cancer. Scores on the Observational Scale of Behavioural Distress (OSBD-R) as well as observer ratings of overall behavioural distress showed that the short story procedure was more effective than either the control condition or the cartoon film in reducing pain and distress.

Specific techniques

In general, materials and techniques that quickly capture and sustain a child's attention are most likely to be effective. Distraction techniques that employ all of the major sensory modalities and require interaction of the child[14] demand a high attentional capacity[4.3] and are more likely to be effective. Novel toys appear to be particularly useful for distracting children, because they provoke curiosity and require children to use their auditory, visual, tactile and/or kinaethestic senses when manoeuvring them. It may be helpful to save the materials that are most likely to distract the child for the procedure itself, rather than using them before the procedure. Alternatively, new materials or activities may be introduced for the procedure. It is extremely important to have a number of materials available so that new ones can be introduced as the child tires of the previous ones. Providing choices can also enhance feelings of control. It is often best to offer a choice from a limited selection (e.g. 'Do you want to look at this book or that book?').

Distraction techniques should be tailored to the developmental level of the child. Younger children (approximately 1 to 6 years of age) will usually need more concrete interventions to capture and sustain their attention. Materials that involve auditory and visual stimulation, such as books with buttons to press for sounds and music, are clinically very effective for children in this age group. The attention of older children may be absorbed by reading a story, or by the 'look and find' books, which require the child to search for hidden pictures. Adolescents (approximately 12 years of age and older) may find listening to music through headphones helpful, and may respond to distraction techniques such as

---

4.3   Attentional capacity is the amount of cognitive attention that is needed to process incoming stimuli.

conversation or joke-telling. Hand-held video games can provide concrete distraction for older children and adolescents, and these games
are useful for decreasing anticipatory distress.

Play therapy

Fundamental principles

Play is a universal element of childhood, and it has existed in all cultures
and in all known historical periods. Play can be a preparation for life via
the realisation of the environment that it can demonstrate, as a repetition of experience and as the communication of symbolic fantasy.
Theories of play emphasise the need for abreaction, for outlets of harmful
impulses, for wish fulfilment, and for a means of enhancing the feeling of
personal value.[15] This may involve the release of extra energy through
imitation, experimentation, assimilation and competition. When considering play it is important to note how useful it is to early ego-strengthening. The child both pretends and tries to master adult situations through
accommodation to external conditions and assimilation of experience
into meaning. Symbolic play is assimilative in that it organises thinking
in terms of symbols and images that have already been partly mastered.
The physical and mental activity that play involves can throw together
ego conflicts, forming a new sense of a basis for the self.

   Play therapy is based on the fact that play is the child's natural
medium of self-expression. It is an opportunity which is given to the
child to 'play out' his or her feelings and problems. Play therapy with
children who have cancer and are undergoing medical procedures has
a threefold purpose.

- It facilitates the child's attempts at mastery of a stressful situation.
- It encourages the expression and verbalisation of emotion.
- It offers the therapist the opportunity to provide information and a
  model for coping with the stresses of cancer treatment in general
  and medical procedures in particular.

Efficacy in acute clinical pain

There is not enough experimental literature to demonstrate the efficacy
of play therapy in the preparation of children with cancer for undergoing
medical procedures, even though clinical experience in many settings

attests to its importance. Puppetry has been shown to be an efficient medium for helping children to cope successfully with illness and hospitalisation, and has been used both to explain medical procedures to children and to encourage feelings of control and mastery during the procedure itself.[16,17] Linn and colleagues[18] used animal puppets in a series of sessions designed primarily to develop the child's sense of mastery. Children were able to express their feelings via the puppets, and to use the puppets to act out their own feelings and also their perceptions of the roles of the doctor, their parents and others. In the work by Linn et al.,[18] sessions focused primarily on themes relating to medical procedures such as bone-marrow aspiration, body integrity, confinement, abandonment and the expressions of rage and fear.

Specific techniques

Play therapy is immediately involving, active and intimate, and it requires neither mobility nor substantial energy. Through play, children frequently express their complex and often confused perceptions of the aetiology and treatment of their illness and their confinement in hospital. A child who acts out several nurses restraining a patient for a procedure is sharing his perception of what happens in the hospital. A child who punishes a toy by sending it to the hospital is demonstrating his feelings about why he is there. In all cases the child's play provides access to issues that are often not being discussed directly.

The play therapy sessions may be structured or unstructured, and should aim to maximise the child's sense of mastery. Children should be given freedom to decide which toys to use and how. Although each session may last as long as 45 minutes or one hour, patients must be given the option of stopping at any time if they wish to do so. Toys selected for the sessions should be easily manipulable so that they do not cause additional frustration for a child whose functioning has been temporarily impaired. Animal toys, rather than toys that represent people, are preferable as they facilitate identification and afford the child more protection than human figures.[19]

If the play therapy involves the administration of medical care, modelling can help children to find ways of coping with their treatment. In response to medical treatments administered by the child, the therapist has the opportunity to ask questions, to cry and to express their anger. However, the therapists' toys always co-operate with the medical staff enacted by the child. In this way children learn acceptable, adaptive, functional ways of handling medical procedures and any other stressful event during their stay in hospital, as well as later in their lives.

Healthcare professionals are constantly being challenged to meet the many needs of their paediatric patients in informed and creative ways. It is important for them to incorporate play as a vital component of their repertoire of 'tools' to promote comfort and alleviate pain and distress.

Case history 4.1

Jennifer was a five-year-old girl with cancer. In one play therapy session she was talking with her doll Barbie as a nurse entered her room. 'You better be good', she whispered to Barbie, 'or she'll give you an injection'. Later in her play she wanted to give an injection to Barbie because she had been a 'naughty girl'. The therapist had to explain to her that she could not perform a procedure on Barbie unless there was a medical reason to do so (i.e. because Barbie was ill). Moreover, only a toy designated as a doctor or nurse could perform the procedure. The unspoken message was that medical procedures are performed for a reason, and that they are not given randomly or as a punishment for misbehaving individuals.

Relaxation

Fundamental principles

'Relaxation training' is a systematic approach to teaching individuals to increase their awareness of their physiological state and achieve a cognitive, emotional and physiological sense of calmness and tranquillity. Relaxation techniques are rarely used on their own in the treatment of procedure-related pain, but rather they are a component of most cognitive–behavioural intervention programmes. There are various forms of relaxation,[20] including the following:

- progressive muscle relaxation[21]
- meditation[22]
- autogenic training[23]
- guided imagery.[24]

Relaxation was first conceived of in the 1930s as a technique for reducing tension and anxiety. Progressive muscle relaxation was first introduced by Jacobson,[21] who found that by extensive practice involving systematic tensing and releasing of muscle groups, anxious patients could learn to discriminate the resulting sensations and produce an experience of deep relaxation. Autogenic training was developed by a psychiatrist from Berlin, Johannes H. Schultz, and was popularised in North America by Luthe.[23] Autogenic training does not require tensing of muscles, but instead involves focusing attention on each muscle group in turn, by suggesting sensations of heaviness and warmth.

The physiology of relaxation

The mechanisms by which relaxation reduces pain are still under investigation, except for a consensus on the obvious mechanism of tension relief. Very little is known about physiological changes in the brain in response to relaxation, but more is known about peripheral physiological change. Even brief progressive muscle relaxation training produces a significant reduction in heart rate, respiratory rate and forearm electromyogram muscle tension.[25] Other documented physiological responses to relaxation include a decrease in oxygen consumption, blood pressure and serum lactic acid levels, an increase in skin resistance, and alterations in blood flow.[26] Plasma norepinephrine levels have been found either to increase or to remain unchanged after relaxation.[27] Increased electroencephalogram alpha- and theta-waves have been reported,[26] but few other brain activity changes have been confirmed as responses to relaxation. One theory maintains that relaxation and meditation result in a shift in hemispheric dominance, with greater activation of centres in the right hemisphere.[26]

Description of techniques

Tension–release relaxation[21]

Progressive muscle relaxation is the most routine of the relaxation techniques. Many people are accustomed to such a high level of tension that they find it difficult to start to relax. Tension–relaxation contrast shows the beginner in relaxation what tension is and how it may be controlled systematically. Since it requires the patient to tense and release muscle groups, it also provides the most feedback to the practitioner on the participation of the patient.

Before beginning the relaxation procedure, the young patient is asked to remove spectacles, toys and books from his or her bed, and wings or hats if they feel uncomfortable. They are then asked to adopt a comfortable body posture, with the arms resting on the arms of the chair, or by the patient's side if he or she is reclining in bed. The arms should lie

flat beside the body, slightly bent at the elbows, and the palms of the
hands should be placed flat on the surface of the bed. The feet should
be uncrossed, and the head and neck should be supported by a pillow
if the patient is lying in bed. The room temperature should be warm
(20–22°C). The lighting should be subdued, telephone calls should be
transferred, and a 'Do not disturb' sign should be placed on the door.
The therapist should remember to turn off his or her beeper. Obviously
these are ideal conditions which are sometime difficult to achieve in a
hospital ward.

The healthcare professional can then say something similar to the
following.

> Relaxation involves learning how to achieve a physical and psycho-
> logical state of calmness in a short period of time, as well as how
> to apply these relaxation skills during medical procedures. You
> may have noticed that when you are under stress (afraid) during a
> medical procedure your body reacts in different ways. Maybe your
> muscles tighten up and become stiff or you sweat a lot or have a
> queasy feeling in your stomach, or maybe you feel your heart race,
> your breathing become short and shallow, or your hands get cold
> and clammy. These are all signals that your body is experiencing
> stress. Through relaxation you will learn how to decrease the
> amount of tension in your body. I suggest that you try to use these
> exercises before you enter the treatment room for the procedure,
> rather than waiting to use them in the middle of the procedure
> when you start feeling pain or fear.
>
> Achieving a state of deep relaxation is a very pleasant experience.
> In addition to reducing pain and fear during medical procedures,
> many children who practise relaxation regularly report feeling a
> greater degree of self-control, less difficulty in falling asleep, and less
> nausea and vomiting when undergoing chemotherapy.
>
> Relaxation training consists of tensing and then relaxing the
> muscles of your body. While you are tensing your muscles, pay
> attention to the muscle sensations and become aware of what it
> feels like for your muscles to be tense. While you are relaxing your
> muscles, pay attention to the muscle sensations and become aware
> of what it feels like for your muscles to be relaxed. Pay special atten-
> tion to the difference between a tense muscle state and a relaxed
> one. Now I want you to close your eyes if you wish and concen-
> trate only on your breathing. ... Now, while you continue to take
> deep, slow relaxing breaths, I want you to turn your attention to
> your hands. First, I'd Iike you to tighten your right hand – that's
> right – hold it tight for about five seconds: 1, 2, 3, 4, 5. Now let it

go, and notice the difference between relaxation and tension. Notice the feeling of ease as you let your hand go. What we'll do now is go through your body alternately tightening and letting go of each muscle group. Let's begin . . .

The therapist should then go over the various muscle groups[4.4] to be tensed, modelling the exercises if necessary to ensure that the patient knows how to tense each muscle group correctly. The 14 muscle groups we usually begin with, and the statements as we go through them with patients, are as follows.

1 *Lower arms and hands.* 'Hold both arms out over your lap and make a fist with each hand'.
2 *Upper arms.* 'Make muscles'.
3 *Calves.* 'Point your toes toward your face as if you were trying to reach your face with your toes (legs stretched)'.
4 *Lower legs.* 'Point your toes away from your face; try to be as long as you can'.
5 *Upper legs.* 'Press your thighs together tightly'.
6 *Stomach.* 'Draw your stomach in tightly, make it disappear as if you were trying to zip up some very tight trousers'.
7 *Chest.* 'Take a deep breath and hold it'.
8 *Shoulders.* 'Draw your shoulders up towards your ears, try to touch your ears with your shoulders'.
9 *Neck.* 'Press your head tightly backward against the pillow (or chair); try to get your head through your pillow'.
10 *Lips.* 'Press your lips together tightly as if you are trying to keep a secret. Do not clamp down with your teeth or bite down on your teeth'.
11 *Eyes.* 'Close your eyes tightly'.
12 *Jaw.* 'Open your mouth as wide as possible as if you were a hungry lion' (an enquiry should have been made about temporomandibular disorder and bruxism before giving this instruction).
13 *Lower forehead.* 'Now I would like you to frown and try to lower your eyebrows'.
14 *Upper forehead.* 'Try to wrinkle your forehead and raise your eyebrows'.

4.4   Although we usually use 14 muscle groups in our first session, it is imperative that the therapist determines whether the patient needs or can benefit from such intense training. Young children who have a short attention span may become bored with such a long procedure. Also children are not usually chronically stressed, and may not need such intensive training. For these individuals we usually begin with an initial session of six or even four muscle groups. The strategy should be individualised to the patient.

Each time, we ask the patient to:

- tighten the muscle group
- hold the tension for approximately 5 seconds
- let the tension go
- notice the difference between tension and relaxation.

Various statements may be inserted during the relaxation phase of the tense–release cycle to encourage relaxation. We vary the combination employed after each cycle so that the patter does not become routine and predictable. As the training progresses, it is not necessary to comment on awareness with each muscle group, but we do mention awareness of the contrasting feelings from time to time. Occasionally, it is helpful to suggest taking a deep breath, holding it and then exhaling while noting the contrast between tension and relaxation.

We complete the exercise by suggesting that the young patient should continue to sit or lie still and enjoy the feelings of relaxation and ease. When he or she wishes, we suggest opening the eyes and returning to the world. At the end of the procedure we ask whether he or she experienced increased tension or anxiety at any time during the relaxation.

Homework.   We instruct the patient to practise relaxation twice daily. A videotape or audiotape of the session can be prepared and given to the patient for home practice, and parents can be trained to coach their children.

During the exercises the therapist should talk in a calm, slow, low-pitched and monotonous voice. It is a good idea to tape-record their voice and experiment with different voices. Novice therapists and children's parents who are being used as coaches should always have a written version of the relaxation procedure in front of them, in order to prevent them from skipping muscle groups, becoming anxious, or forgetting the sequence or correct phrasing of the exercises.

Direct relaxation

One form of direct relaxation is to use the above order of muscle groups and go through them one at a time. However, no tension is used and the young patient simply relaxes each muscle group, one at a time. With practice and experience, relaxation can be as complete without the practised tension. Many young patients prefer this form of relaxation if they find the alternate tensing and loosening tiring and/or boring.

Autogenic relaxation[23]

Autogenics, like direct relaxation, does not require tensing of the muscles first. The focus is on imagining a feeling of warmth and heaviness in each area. The imagery component may relate only to feelings of warmth, heaviness and sensations that accompany relaxation, or it may be augmented at length depending on the will and interest of the patient and the therapist. Imagery creates distraction as well as hypnosis-like experiences of comfort, well-being and mastery of a problem.

Six standard formulas describing specific body sensations constitute the core ingredients of autogenic training (AT). These formulas need to be subvocally repeated by the patient five times before moving on to the next one. In addition, the patient is encouraged to develop personally meaningful images to accompany and enhance the formulas. An important feature that distinguishes AT from both the muscular relaxation technique[28] and meditation[29] is the targeting of specific bodily functions within each of the formulas. The formulas are as follows:

> I am at peace with myself and fully relaxed.
> My right arm is heavy . . . I am at peace.
> My left arm is heavy . . . I am at peace.
> My right leg is heavy . . . I am at peace.
> My left leg is heavy . . . I am at peace.
> My neck and shoulders are heavy . . . I am at peace.
>
> My right arm is warm . . . I am at peace.
> My left arm is warm . . . I am at peace.
> My right leg is warm . . . I am at peace.
> My left leg is warm . . . I am at peace.
> My neck and shoulders are warm . . . I am at peace.
>
> My breathing is calm and regular . . . I am at peace.
> My heartbeat is calm and regular . . . I am at peace.
> My forehead is cool . . . I am at peace.

The patient continues at their own pace, with as much repetition and imagery as they wish. When they are ready to stop, they say to themselves 'When I open my eyes, I will feel refreshed and alert'. They then open their eyes and take a few deep breaths as they stretch and flex their arms and shoulders. They should make sure that they are fully alert and attentive to their environment before they resume their normal activities.

Failure to practise is by far the commonest problem encountered in relaxation training. The practitioner can remind the patient of other learning experiences, such as reading or swimming, in which practice led to mastery.

Meditation

Two similar approaches to meditation have been found to be useful in medical settings. The first involves repeating a phrase or word to oneself, and is known as the *relaxation response*.[30] The second is called *mindfulness meditation*.[31] In the latter, attention is focused not on changing pain perception but on insight developed from distinguishing the sensations as they occur moment by moment. Thoughts about pain are also observed from the position of a neutral observer. Mindfulness meditation has been shown to reduce pain in chronic pain patients.[31] Although relaxation-response training is easy to implement, there are few data available on its effectiveness as a pain reduction method. Box 4.1 summarises the relaxation-response training in simple steps.

Box 4.1:   The relaxation response

1   Choose a focus word or phrase that is rooted in your personal belief system. You will use this word for all of your sessions, so that you will associate it with the calming effect of relaxation.
2   Sit quietly in a comfortable position.
3   Close your eyes.
4   Relax your muscles.
5   Become aware of your breathing, and breathe very slowly and naturally. Simultaneously, repeat your focus word or phrase as you exhale.
6   Continue for 10 to 20 minutes.
7   Practise the technique once or twice daily.

Cognitive therapy

Fundamental principles of the cognitive model

Cognitive therapy is both a philosophical approach to psychotherapy and a strategic combination of techniques for alleviating distress by directly modifying dysfunctional, maladaptive cognitions that are held by the individual who is distressed. The focus in cognitive therapy is on behaviour, emotion, physiological reactions and the individual's cognitions (i.e. thoughts and visual images).[32] The rationale for cognitive therapy is that since a person's cognitions determine their stress reactions to a great extent, modifying negative and maladaptive cognitions is one way in which to reduce their distress.[33]

Cognitive therapy is a structured, time-limited, problem-focused, goal-oriented and educative form of psychotherapy. It is present oriented, emphasises a collaborative therapist–patient relationship, and requires active participation in the treatment by both therapist and patient. In cognitive therapy, patients are taught skills for identifying, evaluating and responding to their dysfunctional thoughts. Techniques for changing mood, behaviour and physiological responses are also employed. The core assumptions of the cognitive model and the fundamental principles of cognitive therapy (*see* Box 4.2) are briefly summarised here because of their relevance to understanding pain as well as psychological approaches to pain management (*see* the reference by Beck for an extended discussion).[34]

Box 4.2:   Fundamental principles of cognitive therapy

- Individuals actively process information.
- Individuals' cognitions and behavioural, emotional and physiological responses are in continuous, dynamic interaction.
- Treatment interventions must be comprehensive and include emotional, physiological, behavioural and cognitive components.
- Individuals must be active participants in treatment if they are to learn adaptive and functional ways of coping with their problems and with life in general.

The core assumptions are as follows.

1   The way in which people construe or interpret events determines how they feel and behave in relation to those events. Thus the way in which a child with cancer construes a medical procedure (painful or not) and related personal events determines how that individual feels and behaves with reference to them.

2   To reduce emotional distress and suffering, psychotherapy encourages individuals to identify and challenge their negative and dysfunctional thinking patterns. Cognitions and emotions are two aspects of the same response (*see* Chapter 1). Emotional reactions, physical sensations (e.g. pain) and behaviours can trigger thoughts, and thoughts

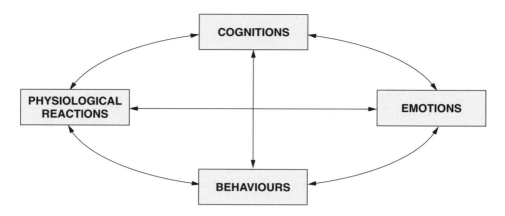

Figure 4.6:   The cognitive model of psychotherapy.

can act as activating events that in turn trigger emotional reactions, physical sensations and particular behaviours, as well as other thoughts (*see* Figure 4.6).

Human beings are active processors of information. They deal with information about what is happening around and within them according to their previous experiences, their expectations, appraisals, mental images and beliefs. According to the cognitive model, the individual's *interpretation* of events – not the events or 'objective reality' as such – influences their behaviours and affective and physiological reactions. Moreover, the way in which a person evaluates and predicts their ability to influence a situation, and the probability and likely consequences of achieving this aim, further shape their perception of an event.[35]

In cognitive psychotherapy, cognitive techniques directly address dysfunctional cognitions, behavioural techniques directly target behaviours, affective techniques directly target emotional experiences, and physiology regulatory techniques directly modify physiological reactions. However, because of the dynamic interaction between these variables, cognitive techniques also address related behaviours, emotional and physiological experiences, and behavioural, affective and physiology regulatory techniques address relevant cognitions.

To summarise, as a model for psychotherapeutic intervention,[36] cognitive therapy seeks to:

- help the patient to identify cognitions that are relevant to their presenting problem
- assist the patient in recognising the integral relationship between cognitions, affects, behaviours and physiological responses

- encourage and support the patient in examining the evidence for and against key beliefs
- encourage and support the patient in the process of trying out an alternative, more functional and adaptive conceptualisation of their problem
- teach the patient to engage in the cognitive disputation process independently of the therapist
- add self-regulatory techniques to the patient's armamentarium.

Efficacy of cognitive therapy in paediatric procedure-related cancer pain

The efficacy of cognitive therapy in paediatric procedure-related cancer pain has been evaluated in a number of clinical trials, which are reviewed briefly below.

Jay and colleagues[37,38] developed a multicomponent intervention 'package' of cognitive–behavioural techniques (CBT) designed to teach effective coping skills and to reduce children's distress during bone-marrow aspirations and lumbar punctures. The intervention package consists of five primary components, namely filmed modelling, incentive, breathing exercises, emotive imagery and distraction, and behavioural rehearsal. Patients are first shown an 11-minute film of another child undergoing a bone-marrow aspiration or lumbar puncture. In this film, the child narrates the steps of the medical procedure together with their thoughts and feelings at critical points, and models positive coping behaviours (breathing exercises, imagery) and positive 'self-statements' (e.g. 'I know I can do it') during the medical procedure. Since research[39] supports the superiority of modelling that is based on coping, as opposed to mastery models, the child in the film exhibits a realistic amount of anxiety (e.g. 'I am a little scared') but then copes effectively, as opposed to not exhibiting any anxiety or distress. After the film, patients are taught a simple breathing exercise. Each child is instructed to take a deep breath and to let it out slowly while making a hissing sound ('s-s-s').[40] This serves as an attention-distraction technique and gives the child something active to do during the procedure, rather than merely passively submitting to it.

The incentive component involves showing the child a small trophy. The latter is presented to the child as a symbol of mastery, and children can obtain the trophy if they do 'the best that they could possibly do'. Each child is encouraged to lie still (which reduces the likelihood of complications when performing the medical procedure) and practise their breathing exercises (which generally preclude severe behavioural distress, such as kicking and screaming). The purpose of the trophies is to try to transform the meaning of pain for the child. Rather than perceiving the bone-marrow aspiration or lumbar puncture as a distressing, punitive event, the idea is to try to persuade children to view it as a challenge, and as an opportunity to master a difficult situation, thus resulting in positive feelings of self-efficacy and increased self-esteem.

Emotive imagery is a technique that involves ascertaining a child's superhero or fantasy images and then weaving these images into the current medical situation. For instance, a young child may wish to imagine that he is Superman's agent, and that Superman has asked him to undergo the medical procedure as part of a special mission. Such images presumably transform the meaning of the pain for the child and provide another distraction technique. The final component of the package is behavioural rehearsal. In this phase the child is encouraged to 'play doctor' and to give a doll the bone-marrow aspiration or lumbar puncture using actual medical equipment (with older children, this is called a demonstration). The rehearsal provides information for the child and allows him or her to prepare mentally and emotionally for the impending medical procedure.

Jay and colleagues conducted a series of studies that systematically examined distress behaviour, antecedent variables, and the effects of behavioural and pharmacological interventions on procedural distress. In their first study,[37] five children aged 3–7 years, who had been referred for severe anxiety and behavioural distress related to bone-marrow aspirations and lumbar punctures, reduced their distress scores after intervention by at least 50%.

The second study[38] was a comparison of the CBT package with oral diazepam and an attention-control condition (30 minutes of cartoon watching prior to the bone-marrow aspiration) delivered in the context of a repeated-measures, counterbalanced design. A total of 56 children with leukaemia, aged 3–13 years, were studied. The dependent variables were scores on the Observational Scale of Behavioural Distress (OSBD), self-reported pain, and pulse and blood pressure readings. Overall, children in the CBT group had significantly lower pain ratings, OSBD scores, and pulse rates compared with either the diazepam group or the attention-control group. Diazepam was useful for lowering anticipatory distress, but had no effect on distress during the procedure (encounter phase). In fact, there was no difference in OSBD scores in the different treatment groups when the encounter phase of the bone-marrow aspiration was analysed separately.

The next study[41] investigated the combined effects of oral diazepam and CBT. Within a repeated-measures factorial design, 83 children aged 3.5

to 12 years were assigned to either CBT or a combination of CBT plus diazepam. Dependent variables included observed behavioural distresses measured by the OSBD, self-reported pain and anxiety, and pulse rate. Both groups showed a decrease in their OSBD and self-reported pain scores between baseline and intervention. However, the CBT plus diazepam group showed only one-third of the reduction that was observed in children in the CBT-only group. The investigators suggested that the diazepam might have interfered with the learning of CBT strategies. In addition, the children may have been unable to remain focused on the imagery and distraction tasks during the procedure due to the effects of diazepam.

The last study[42] was an interesting comparison of CBT with general anaesthesia (GA) in alleviating the distress of 18 paediatric cancer patients (aged 3 to 12 years) undergoing bone-marrow aspirations. CBT and short-acting mask anaesthesia were delivered within a repeated-measures, counterbalanced design and subjects were randomly assigned to one of two sequence orders. The results indicated that children exhibited more behavioural distress in the CBT condition for the first minute of lying down on the treatment table. With regard to the child outcome measures, no significant differences in self-reported pain and fear, pulse or anticipation of the next bone-marrow aspiration were found in relation to CBT vs. general anaesthesia. The data collected with regard to parental stress and coping also demonstrated virtually no differences between CBT and GA. However, parents rated significantly more behavioural adjustment symptoms 24 hours after the bone-marrow aspiration when their children had received general anaesthesia. No differences were found in children's and parents' preference for CBT vs. general anaesthesia.

Kazak and colleagues[43,44] used a number of the same CBT components to compare the efficacy of conscious sedation with a combination of conscious sedation and psychological intervention for children undergoing bone-marrow aspirations and lumbar punctures. In a randomised, controlled prospective trial of 92 children with leukaemia, the combined treatment was found to be superior to conscious sedation alone on ratings of child distress by mothers and nurses. When compared with a cross-sectional control group consisting of the parents of 70 patients in first remission prior to the prospective study, the combined intervention group showed lower levels of child distress. The data also showed decreases in distress over time, and concurrent improvements in quality of life and parental stress, and supported an inverse association between distress and age of the child.

Clearly, CBT has been shown in a number of studies (summarised in Table 4.1) to reduce the distress of children with cancer undergoing a variety of painful medical procedures, and it is now considered to be

Table 4.1: Comparison of cognitive–behavioural intervention studies for paediatric procedure-related cancer pain

Study	Patients (n)	Age range (years)	Design	Interventions	Outcome measures	Results
Jay et al.[37]	5	3–7	Baseline post-treatment	CBT	Observed distress (OSBD)	50% reduction in OSBD scores after intervention
Jay et al.[38]	56	3–13	Repeated measures, counterbalanced	Oral diazepam Attention control (30 minutes of cartoon watching) prior to bone-marrow aspiration	Self-reported pain, observed distress (OSBD), pulse, blood pressure	Patients had significantly lower pain and OSBD scores and pulse rates in the CBT condition, compared with either the diazepam or the attention-control group
Jay et al.[41]	83	3.5–12	Repeated measures, factorial	CBT CBT plus diazepam	Self-reported pain, self-reported fear, observed distress (OSBD), pulse	No significant group differences for any of the dependent variables
Jay et al.[42]	18	3–12	Repeated measures, counterbalanced	CBT General anaesthesia	Self-reported pain, self-reported fear, observed distress (OSBD), pulse, PPQ, a number of parent and nurse assessment measures	No significant differences in self-reported pain and fear, pulse or anticipation of the next bone-marrow aspiration between CBT and anaesthesia Patients exhibited more behavioural distress in the CBT condition for the first minute of lying down on the treatment table No differences in children's and parents' preference for CBT vs. anaesthesia

| Kazak et al.[43,44] | 92 + 70 | <18 | Parallel group plus cross-sectional control group | Conscious sedation (midazolam + morphine)
Conscious sedation (midazolam + morphine) plus distraction (play, imagery, counting, breathing)
Cross-sectional control group | PPQ Parent Stress Index. Paediatric Quality of Life Scale, parent and staff ratings of child distress, parent self-rating of stress, staff rating of parent distress | Significant differences between groups according to child distress ratings of parents and staff |

Source: Adapted from Ellis and Spanos (1994) Cognitive behavioural interventions for children's distress during bone-marrow aspirations and lumbar punctures: a critical review. *J Pain Symptom Manage*. 9: 96–108.
CBT, cognitive–behavioural therapy; OSBD: Observational Scale of Behavioural Distress; PPQ: Perception of Procedures Questionnaire.

a well-established treatment in the management of procedure-related pain.[45] A Consensus Conference on the Management of Pain in Childhood Cancer recommended that cognitive interventions should be a routine part of the management of painful procedures.[46]

McCarthy and colleagues[47] surveyed 15 paediatric bone-marrow transplant units and 32 paediatric haematology/oncology centres in the USA with regard to the use and effectiveness of cognitive–behavioural interventions and the availability of support services. The results indicated that most centres (88%) use a number of cognitive–behavioural interventions to help children to cope with painful procedures. However, some interventions, such as providing information before procedures and positive reinforcement, were used more frequently than more complex interventions. In general, nurses were the major providers of these interventions, which suggests that nurses need to continue to study appropriate ways to incorporate the use of effective psychological interventions into the routine care of children with cancer.

Cognitive therapy for acute paediatric pain: the techniques

Building from the foundation of the cognitive therapy model of Beck,[36] Beck and colleagues,[48] and Turk *et al.*'s treatment model for chronic pain,[35] cognitive therapy for acute paediatric pain is guided by the idea that it is crucial to translate vague complaints, distress and fears into more specific and concrete terms that are amenable to therapeutic interventions. Young cancer patients in pain are provided with information about pain mechanisms and are exposed to the cognitive model of pain management. The therapy is self-help oriented, and is aimed at teaching patients skills for identifying, evaluating and responding to their dysfunctional thoughts. Patients are also taught behavioural coping skills (e.g. pacing and shaping) and physiology regulatory skills (e.g. relaxation techniques).

The emphasis is on equipping the young patient with strategies for coping with different stressful situations during cancer treatment. Patients are coached in the use of positive self-statements at each phase of a painful procedure, and are taught how to identify and cognitively challenge negative self-talk that could lead to depression, anxiety and fear. The programme also includes psychosocial and interpersonal interventions to address and modify the role of parents in the maintenance of a child's pain-related distress.

The ultimate aim of cognitive therapy for pain management is to promote cognitive restructuring, which involves a reorganisation of the person's thinking, emotions, behaviours and physiological reactions with regard to pain, and promotes the realisation that pain management and pain relief are possible and attainable, and that medical procedures are not necessarily a source of enormous distress. Thinking can sabotage or foster the success of any pain treatment, including pharmacological or psychological interventions.

The four core components of cognitive therapy for children undergoing invasive medical procedures are as follows:

- education
- skills acquisition
- cognitive and behavioural rehearsal
- generalisation and maintenance.

These will be described briefly in turn below.

Patient education

The first priority in the intervention programme is to build rapport, mutual trust and respect, and to educate the young patient about the close interrelationship between thoughts, emotions, behaviours and physiological reactions. Establishing a rationale for psychological techniques is critical. We almost always provide our patients with information about pain mechanisms in general, and about procedure-related pain in particular, in terms that they can understand. A simplified explanation of the gate control theory of pain is a good way to begin to introduce the notion that psychological as well as physiological factors play a role in determining how pain is experienced. This concept can be made personally relevant to patients if the therapist helps them to identify factors that increase or decrease their experience of pain, discussing these in terms of opening or closing the 'pain gate'. An example constructed by Charles, a 6-year-old boy undergoing lumbar punctures, is provided in Table 4.2.

Table 4.2:   A young patient's understanding of what determines the intensity of his pain

More pain	Less pain
Fear	Medicines
Anxiety	Mum
Tension	Relaxing
Fighting the nurse	Laughing
Worrying	Thinking of something else

Skills acquisition

In this phase, the patient is helped to identify and evaluate their existing strategies for coping with pain, and to develop more effective ones. Functional and adaptive coping strategies that can be used by young cancer patients include the following:

- *distraction* (e.g. doing mental arithmetic and spelling, engaging in a pleasant fantasy, thinking about engaging in a pleasant activity, focusing on an object in the treatment room, focusing on squeezing the nurse's hand)
- *positive affirmations* (e.g. verbalising positive and encouraging self-statements, such as 'Stay calm', 'I can cope with the procedure', 'It will soon be over', 'Practise your coping skills')
- *relaxation* (e.g. deep breathing, progressive muscle relaxation, autogenic relaxation)
- *pain relief, replacement and transformational imagery* (e.g. imagining the painful area becoming numb, imagining receiving an anaesthetic injection to the painful area, imagining oneself floating, imagining oneself experiencing the pain in a different context, such as that of a spy or superhero).
- *decatastrophising dysfunctional beliefs* (i.e. helping patients to realise that a medical procedure is really not as awful as they thought or imagined)
- *cognitive restructuring* – in cognitive restructuring the therapist assesses the patient's automatic thoughts associated with their fears, sense of helplessness and anger before, during and after a procedure. It helps them to identify any irrational thoughts that they may have. Dysfunctional thoughts are subjected to examination, and are then refuted, reframed, reinterpreted and replaced with more realistic thoughts. Patients are also taught to do this on their own (*see* Box 4.4).

Case history 4.2

Maria was a 15-year-old girl with Hodgkin's lymphoma. Every time she was about to undergo any procedure, painful or not, her automatic thought was 'I cannot take this any more'. She was taught to examine this and similar thoughts and to develop more accurate and adaptive ones. For example, 'Is it really true that I cannot deal with this? No. It may be difficult, but I've done it before and I can do it again'.

Patients typically need much help in fully describing their thoughts and feelings. They may say that they simply felt anxious, and do not mention any thoughts that would lead to feelings of anxiety (*see* Box 4.3). In this case the therapist should help the patient to reconstruct the thought which was associated with that feeling. Only when patients can readily identify automatic thoughts and feelings should the therapist move on to instruct them in evaluating the accuracy of negative thoughts and generating alternative thoughts (*see* Box 4.4).

Box 4.3:   The various components of lumbar puncture-related pain as constructed by a 12-year-old girl with non-Hodgkin's lymphoma

Physiological reactions	My palms become sweaty when I am in pain, my heart pounds, sometimes I feel dizzy or faint, I am breathing fast and I feel pressure in my chest. I cannot stay relaxed when I hurt
Cognitions	I feel disoriented and confused when I hurt, and I think about the pain constantly. During painful procedures it is difficult for me to think of anything besides the pain. I worry when I am in pain
Emotions	I dread feeling pain. When pain comes on strong, I think that I might become paralysed. I think that if my pain goes on like this, it will never decrease
Behaviours	When I feel pain I try to stay as still as possible, but usually I end up crying, resisting and fighting the nurse

---

Box 4.4:   Cognitive restructuring
- The therapist provides the young patient with a rationale for challenging negative automatic thoughts.
- The therapist and patient systematically identify and challenge the evidence that supports or refutes specific automatic thoughts.
- The therapist and patient develop alternative, more accurate, functional and adaptive thoughts.

Cognitive and behavioural rehearsal

After learning different skills, patients are asked to use them in imaginal situations in the therapist's office. They are asked to imagine themselves in the treatment room undergoing a procedure, and to visualise themselves employing their relaxation and cognitive coping skills in those situations.[49] The therapist can guide the young patient through the mental rehearsal of the painful procedure and say something like the following.

Close your eyes and imagine that in an hour you are about to undergo a lumbar puncture. Prepare yourself. Remind yourself of the coping techniques that you can employ as the stress and pain begin to increase. What can you say to yourself at this point? What do you do with your body? (Wait for the patient to answer.) After the doctor has cleansed your back and is about to insert the needle, you begin to employ appropriate coping techniques such as controlling your breathing, relaxing your muscles, talking to yourself in a positive way, distracting yourself in some way, and thinking of something that takes your mind off the pain. The needle is in and you feel a stinging pain. You cope with it! What can you say to yourself and do to your body to help you to cope once the pain has started? (Wait for an answer.) If things are not going well and the doctor needs to try again, you must be ready to employ your most powerful coping techniques. What can you say to remind yourself to use your most powerful coping strategies? The procedure has finished. At this point, you want to remind yourself that you got through the pain, and you want to give yourself credit that you handled it well. What can you say to yourself to give yourself credit for handling the situation well? (Wait for the patient to answer.)

In order to review and consolidate the training procedures, the patient may be asked to role play a situation in which the therapist and the patient reverse roles. The patient is instructed that it will be their job to assume the role of a new patient who has not received any cognitive–behavioural training. This role-reversal exercise is employed because research on attitude change indicates that when people have to improvise, as in a role-playing situation, they generate exactly the types of arguments that are most convincing.[35] Such role playing also provides the therapist with a means of assessing any conflicting thoughts, feelings or doubts that the patient may have.

Generalisation and maintenance

The purpose of the generalisation and maintenance phase is to help young patients to transfer the skills learned in the office to the actual treatment room, and to retain their learned skills throughout the course of their cancer treatment. During this phase the therapist provides patients with the realistic expectation that setbacks may occur, and that these setbacks should not be regarded as evidence of failure, but rather instead they should be viewed as cues to use their coping skills more consistently. Moreover, during this phase patients are provided with tangible evidence of the progress they have made during treatment. This encourages them to maintain the belief that their personal efforts have contributed to their improvement, and that they are capable of facing future challenges effectively. This evidence can be provided either by videotaping the patient during a procedure before and after cognitive therapy, or by showing them the scoring of their pain before and after the intervention.

Family involvement and attitudes

If family members are active in the patient's care during cancer treatment, their beliefs and attitudes need to be considered, as they can assist or hinder the process of therapy. Ideally, family members support the use of analgesic methods, whether these are pharmacological or psychological. Some families may actively discourage interested patients from trying different approaches, or may convey all of their own fears about these approaches (e.g. a parent who is terrified of general anaesthesia may turn a safe and effective intervention into a fearful and potentially lethal one in their child's mind). When family members are supportive and available, they may be good 'coaches' for patients, helping them to use psychological interventions when the clinician is not available, and encouraging their child to comply fully with pharmacological interventions and to co-operate with medical and nursing personnel.

Case history 4.3

Johnny was a 5-year-old boy with acute myeloid leukaemia. He was undergoing bone-marrow aspirations under general anaesthesia, and was taught cognitive therapy for lumbar punctures and venepunctures which were performed under a local anaesthetic. A cognitive assessment of his concerns with regard to medical procedures revealed cognitions of the following nature: 'My back will break' (during a lumbar puncture), 'The procedure will never end', a visual image of a 'huge needle' and 'I have been a bad boy recently (kicking my big brother and swearing at and pinching my baby sister) – that is why I have to have all these injections and pain'. He also displayed feelings such as fear, anxiety and anger before and during medical procedures, physiological reactions such as muscle tension and increased heart rate ('my heart beats so fast it will explode'), and behaviours such as resistance, screaming and crying. After a comprehensive psychological assessment, Johnny was provided with information about how pain works, and he was taught breathing techniques and relaxation and his major negative automatic thoughts were challenged. An example of the cognitive techniques used is given below.

Therapist: 'What is your worst fear during the spinal tap? What do you think will happen?'

Johnny: 'The nurse squeezes me so hard that she will break my back'.

Therapist: 'Almost all of the children in the ward undergo spinal taps often. How many have you seen walking around with broken backs?'

Johnny: (Reluctantly) '. . . none'.

Therapist: 'Why do you think that is? Could it be that we are hiding them from you? That the children with broken backs only come out at night?'

Johnny: 'Noooh. I would know it if some of my friends had broken backs. Mummy would have told me as well'.

Therapist: 'Good, so that means that no child has suffered a broken back as a result of a spinal tap'.

Johnny: 'Yeah' (with a smile).

Therapist: 'Have you noticed when the nurse squeezes you most? Does she say anything at that time?'

Johnny: 'She says "Stand still, just relax and be curled up" '.

Therapist: 'And do you do that?'

Johnny: 'Yep'.

Therapist: 'Really? Do you do as the nurse says?'

Johnny: (reluctantly) 'No . . . I fight with her most of the time, and she squeezes me harder! Sometimes she says "if you do not stay still we will have to give you GA" '.

Therapist: 'So, what do you think you can do next time so that the nurse squeezes you less?'

Johnny: 'Not to go to the treatment room!'

Therapist: 'That is one possibility, but as we have discussed on previous occasions, you need to have LPs and VPs. Remember?'

Johnny: 'Yeah. Well, I could relax, stand still, curled up and not fight with the nurse!'

Therapist: 'Do you think you can do that?'

Johnny: 'Yeah'.

Therapist: 'OK. We will talk later about what specifically you can do so that you can remain relaxed and curled up during the LP. Would you like to tell me now what else scares you in the spinal tap?'

Johnny: 'This huge needle!'

Therapist: 'Huge? How big do you think the needle is?'

Johnny: 'That big' (stretches his arms as far as he can).

Therapist: 'Wow! That is really big. Are you sure it is that big?'

Johnny: (reluctantly) 'Yeah'.

Therapist: 'Have you ever actually seen the needle?'

Johnny: 'No'.

Therapist: 'Where do you think doctors keep the needles? Do you know? I don't think we have a cupboard big enough in the ward to keep such a big needle. Maybe they keep it in the wardrobe!'

Johnny: 'No, silly! You cannot keep a needle in the wardrobe. They put all the needles together in the autoclave and sterilise them. Come – I'll show you!'

The patient led the therapist to the treatment room where they met Dr Helen. There they saw the needles, and the doctor further explained to Johnny the importance of remaining still and calm during the procedure, and gave him a demonstration of how she actually performs a lumbar puncture on a doll. The challenging of the automatic negative thoughts continued for three sessions until Johnny had completed his programme and had a realistic appreciation of what a lumbar puncture and a venepuncture involve. He also decided which coping statements to use during the procedures. These included 'I can do it', 'Pain will go away soon', 'I am almost there' and 'I am a brave warrior'. After four sessions Johnny was able to undergo lumbar punctures and venepunctures easily, and was glad that he did not have to fast for a general anaesthetic for lumbar puncture. He was proudly describing his accomplishment to his brother and grandparents, and he was 'awarded' the title of the psychologist's 'assistant', with responsibilities to demonstrate the techniques to other children in the ward and to introduce the approach to new members of staff.

References

1 Siegel LJ (1976) Preparation of children for hospitalization: a selected review of the research literature. *J Pediatr Psychol.* **1**: 26–30.

2 Schechter NL (1985) Pain and pain control in children. *Curr Prob in Pediatr.* **15**: 1–67.

3 Anderson K and Masur FT (1983) Psychological preparation for invasive medical and dental procedures. *Behav Med.* **6**: 1–8.

4 Zeltzer L, Altman A, Cohen D, LeBaron S, Maunskela E and Schechter N (1990) American Academy of Pediatrics: Report of the Subcommittee on the Management of Pain Associated with Procedures in Children with Cancer. *Pediatrics.* **86**: 826–31.

5 Liossi C (1999) Management of pediatric procedure-related cancer pain. *Pain Rev.* **6**: 279–302.

6 Fowler-Kerry S and Lander JR (1987) Management of injection pain in children. *Pain.* **30**: 169–75.

7 Smith KE, Ackerson JP, Blotcky AD and Berkow R (1990) Preferred coping styles of pediatric cancer patients during invasive medical procedures. *J Psychosoc Oncol.* **8**: 59–70.

8 Blount RL, Bachanes PJ, Powers SW *et al.* (1991) Training children to cope and parents to coach them during routine examinations: effects on child, parent and staff behaviors. *Behav Ther.* **23**: 689–706.

9   Gonzalez JC, Routh DK, Saab PG *et al.* (1989) Effects of parent presence on children's reactions to injections: behavioral, physiological and subjective aspects. *J Pediatr Psychol.* **14**: 449–62.

10 Powers SW, Blount RL, Bachanas PJ, Cotter MW and Swan S (1993) Helping preschool leukemia patients and their parents cope during injections. *J Pediatr Psychol.* **18**: 681–95.

11 Cohen LL, Blount RL and Panopoulos G (1997) Nurse coaching and cartoon distraction: an effective and practical intervention to reduce child parent and nurse distress during immunizations. *J Pediatr Psychol.* **22**: 355–70.

12 Vessey JA, Carlson KL and McGill J (1994) Use of distraction with children during an acute pain experience. *Nurs Res.* **43**(6): 369–72.

13 Mason S, Johnson MH and Wooley C (1999) A comparison of distractors for controlling distress in young children during medical procedures. *J Clin Psychol Med Settings.* **6**: 239–48.

14 Bush JP, Melamed BG, Sheras PL and Greenbaum PE (1986) Mother–child patterns of coping with anticipatory medical stress. *Health Psychol.* **5**: 137–57.

15 Axline V (1989) *Play Therapy.* Churchill Livingstone, Edinburgh.

16 Linn S (1978) Puppet therapy in hospitals: helping children cope. *JAMWA.* **33**: 61–5.

17 Hodges C (1998) Easing children's pain. *Nurs Times.* **94**(10): 55–6, 58.

18 Linn S, Beardslee W and Patenaude AF (1986) Puppet therapy in pediatric bone-marrow transplant patients. *J Pediatr Psychol.* **11**: 37–46.

19 Walker C (1989) Use of art and play therapy in pediatric oncology. *J Pediatr Oncol Nurs.* **6**: 121–6.

20 Smith JC (1990) *Cognitive–Behavioral Relaxation Training: a new system of strategies for treatment and assessment.* Springer, New York.

21 Jacobson E (1974) *Progressive Relaxation.* University of Chicago Press, Chicago.

22 Lichstein KL (1988) *Clinical Relaxation Strategies.* John Wiley & Sons, New York.

23 Luthe W (1963) Autogenic training: method, research and application in medicine. *Am J Psychother.* **17**: 174.

24 Bellack A (1973) Reciprocal inhibition of a laboratory-conditioned fear. *Behav Res Ther.* **11**: 11–18.

25 Blumenstein B, Bar-Eli M and Tenenbaum G (1995) The augmenting role of biofeedback: effects of autogenic imagery and music training on physiological indices and athletic performance. *J Sports Sci.* **13**: 343–54.

26 Muck-Weymann M, Tritt K, Hornstein OP, Mosler T and Joraschky P (1998) Rhythmical changes of the cutaneous blood flow in the forehead region under the condition of hypnoid relaxation. *Vasa.* **27**: 220–23.

27 Infante JR, Torres-Avisbal M, Pinel P *et al.* (2001) Catecholamine levels in practitioners of the transcendental meditation. *Physiol Behav.* **72**: 141–6.

28 Jacobson E (1938, reprinted in 1974) *Progressive Relaxation.* University of Chicago Press, Chicago.

29 Mishima N, Kubota S and Nagata S (1999) Psychophysiological correlates of relaxation induced by standard autogenic training. *Psychother Psychosom.* **68**: 207–13.

30 Manocha R. (2000) Why meditation? *Aust Fam Physician.* **29**: 1135–8.

31 Dunn BR, Hartigan JA and Mikulas WL (1999) Concentration and mindfulness meditations: unique forms of consciousness? *Appl Psychophysiol Biofeedback.* **24**: 147–65.

32 Meichenbaum D and Turk D (1976) The cognitive–behavioral management of anxiety, anger and pain. In: P O Davidson (ed.) *The Behavioral Management of Anxiety, Depression and Pain.* Brunner/Mazel, New York, 1–34.

33 Meichenbaum DH (1977) *Cognitive Behavior Modification: an integrative approach.* Plenum, New York.

34 Beck JS (1995) *Cognitive Therapy: basics and beyond.* Guilford Press, New York.

35 Turk DC, Meichenbaum D and Genest M (1983) *Pain and Behavioral Medicine: a cognitive behavioral perspective.* Guilford Press, New York.

36 Beck AT (1976) *Cognitive Therapy and the Emotional Disorders.* International Universities Press, New York.

37 Jay SM, Elliott CH, Ozolins M and Pruitt C (1985) Behavioural management of children's distress during painful medical procedures. *Behav Res Ther.* **23**: 513–20.

38 Jay SM, Elliott CH, Katz ER and Siegel SE (1987) Cognitive–behavioural and pharmacologic interventions for children undergoing painful medical procedures. *J Consult Clin Psychol.* **55**: 860–65.

39 Meichenbaum D and Jaremko M (1983) *Stress Reduction and Prevention.* Plenum Press, New York.

40 Elliott CH and Olson RA (1983) The management of children's distress in response to painful medical treatment for burn injuries. *Behav Res Ther.* **21**: 675–83.

41 Jay SM, Elliott CH, Woody P and Siegel SE (1991) An investigation of cognitive–behaviour therapy combined with oral valium for children undergoing painful medical procedures. *Health Psychol.* **10**: 317–22.

42 Jay SM, Elliott CH, Fitzgibbons I, Woody P and Siegel S (1995) A comparative study of cognitive behaviour therapy versus general anaesthesia for children undergoing painful medical procedures. *Pain.* **62**: 3–9.

43 Kazak AE, Penati B, Brophy P and Himelstein B (1998) Pharmacologic and psychologic interventions for procedural pain. *Pediatrics.* **1**: 59–66.

44 Kazak AE, Penati B, Boyer BA *et al.* (1996) A randomized controlled prospective study of a psychological and pharmacological intervention protocol for procedural distress in pediatric leukemia. *J Pediatr Psychol.* **21**: 615–31.

45 Powers SW (1999) Empirically supported treatments in pediatric psychology: procedure-related pain. *J Pediatr Psychol.* **24**: 131–45.

46 Pain Management Guideline Panel (1992) *Acute Pain Management: operative or medical procedures and trauma. Guideline report.* Agency for Health Care Policy and Research, Rockville, MD.

47 McCarthy AM, Cool VA, Petersen M and Bruene DA (1996) Cognitive behavioral pain and anxiety interventions in pediatric oncology centers and bone-marrow transplant units. *J Pediatr Oncol Nurs.* **13**: 3–12.

48 Beck AT, Rush AJ, Shaw BR and Emery G (1979) *Cognitive Therapy of Depression.* Guilford Press, New York.

49 Gatchel R and Turk D (1996) *Psychological Treatment for Pain: a practitioner's handbook.* Guilford Press, New York.

5

The psychological management of paediatric procedure-related cancer pain. Part 2

Christina Liossi

Introduction

Hypnosis is among the oldest and best-documented psychological treatments for pain. From the controversial reports of its use in surgery prior to the development of chemo-anaesthesia,[1] to the extensive experimental and clinical literature on its use during the last 30 years,[2] hypnosis has been observed to provide almost total relief from the sensation of pain in some individuals. Hypnosis is one of the most empirically tested psychological interventions in the management of procedure-related pain, especially pain due to lumbar punctures and bone-marrow aspirations, and has acquired status as an empirically supported intervention.[3] The purpose of this chapter is to review the use of hypnosis in children with cancer. First, hypnosis is defined and current theories about it are delineated. This discussion is followed by a brief description of the current body of knowledge with regard to hypnotic responsiveness. Next there is a comprehensive review of hypnotic interventions for pain associated with paediatric procedures, and the chapter concludes with a discussion of the actual hypnotic techniques that can be used to help children with cancer to undergo painful procedures with minimal pain and distress.

Fundamental principles

Defining hypnosis

Hypnosis is a term that is used in very different ways by different theorists, researchers and clinicians. Many attempts have been made to define hypnosis, both in terms of the phenomena involved and in terms of possible causal mechanisms, but no definition has yet satisfactorily answered all of the questions raised by the subject matter. The term has so many different connotations (e.g. altered state, loss of will, enhanced abilities) that any attempt to define it is bound to have drawbacks and limitations. Controversy about the nature of hypnosis and its utility as a construct has existed since the phenomenon was first described.

Given the contentious nature of the field, the American Psychological Association, Division of Psychological Hypnosis (Division 30) prepared the following definition and description of hypnosis

> Hypnosis is a procedure during which a health professional or researcher suggests that a client, patient or subject experience changes in sensation, perception, thought or behaviour. The hypnotic context is generally established by an induction procedure. Although there are many different hypnotic inductions, most include suggestions for relaxation, calmness and well-being. Instruction to imagine or think about pleasant experiences is also commonly included in hypnotic inductions.
>
> People respond to hypnosis in different ways. Some describe their experiences as an altered state of consciousness. Others describe hypnosis as a normal state of focused attention, in which they feel very calm and relaxed. Regardless of how and to what degree they respond, most people describe the experience as very pleasant.
>
> Some people are very responsive to hypnotic suggestion, and others are less responsive. A person's ability to experience hypnotic suggestion can be inhibited by fears and concerns arising from some common misconceptions. Contrary to some depictions of hypnosis in books, movies or on television, people who have been hypnotised do not lose control over their behaviour. They typically remain aware of who they are and where they are, and unless amnesia has been specifically suggested, they usually remember what transpired during hypnosis. Hypnosis makes it easier for people to experience suggestions, but it does not force them to have those experiences.[4]

Current theories of hypnosis

From the observations on the uses to which hypnosis and hypnotic phenomena have been put, various theories concerning the fundamentals of hypnosis have been proposed. In the past, the majority of hypnosis researchers believed that there is an hypnotic state which differs fundamentally from the waking state.[5] This postulated state was assumed to be the 'essence' of hypnosis[6] and its definition. The state debate began when Sarbin[7] and Barber[8] rejected the idea that hypnotic responses were due to an altered state of consciousness. They maintained that all of the hypnotic phenomena could be accounted for without postulating any special state or condition. From their perspective, hypnotic behaviours are like other complex social behaviours – they are a product of factors such as ability, attitude, belief, expectancy, attribution and interpretation of the situation.

Nowadays, according to Kirsch and Lynn,[9] instead of two opposing camps, there is a continuum of positions on the issue. At one end of this continuum are those who support the concept of *hypnotic state* in its strongest possible form, as a condition that is fundamentally different both to normal waking consciousness and to other altered states, such as daydreaming and relaxation. These include Ericksonian and contemporary psychoanalytical theorists.[10,11] At the other end of the continuum are theorists who use the term *state* to describe hypnotic phenomena but who deny that it explains or causes those phenomena in any way,[12,13] those who acknowledge allegiance to the state construct but then ignore it entirely in their theories of hypnotic responding,[14,15] and those who explicitly reject the hypnotic state construct as inaccurate and misleading.[16–23]

Like the state issue, the trait issue can most accurately be portrayed as a continuum rather than as a dichotomy.[9] Most scholars recognise a role for stable individual differences and a role for contextual variables in determining hypnotic response. Furthermore, most of them emphasise the importance of considering the interaction between these variables.[17,21,23,24] They differ with regard to the relative emphasis that should be placed on these two types of variables. Overall, a person's receptivity to utilising hypnosis as a window of opportunity for pain relief depends on factors such as motivation, beliefs and hypnotic capacity.

Hypnotic responsiveness in children

The fact that individuals differ in the degree to which they respond to hypnosis and to hypnotic suggestions is obvious to anyone who has worked in this area. Several studies have demonstrated that children are more hypnotically responsive than adults.[25,26] As Olness and Gardner[27] noted, hypnotic ability is limited in children below the age of 3 years, reaches a peak during middle childhood (7–14 years), and then decreases in adolescence, remaining stable through to midlife before it decreases again in the older population. There are no significant differences in hypnotic responsiveness between boys and girls at any age.

Hypnotic responsiveness scales are used to measure an individual's hypnotic ability.[28] The advantages of these instruments are that they permit the assessment of a broad range of hypnotic behaviours, they require relatively little time to administer, score and interpret, they facilitate the collection of normative data, and they are readily quantifiable. Today the most commonly used measure for children is the Stanford Hypnotic Clinical Scale for Children (SHCS-Children), which is a 7-item, 20-minute scale that is administered to subjects individually. SHCS-Children scores are based on the assessment of both behaviour and experience (via verbal reports), and range from 0 to 7.

Childhood hypnotic responsiveness and treatment outcome

There is a consistent finding that highly hypnotisable subjects experience a greater decrease in pain than less hypnotisable subjects in laboratory studies,[29,30] but even in this case hypnotisability is not the best predictor of response.[31] For clinical patients, with stronger motivating factors, the response on standard measures seems to be even less useful as a predictor of ability to benefit from these strategies.[32,33]

Although there are conflicting and inconsistent clinical and laboratory reports with regard to who is or is not a good candidate for hypnosis, clinical experience attests to the fact that almost any patient can benefit from individualised treatment, so long as they want to use hypnosis. With some motivation on the part of the patient and with individualisation of the methods, nearly any child with cancer can benefit from these techniques, although more responsive patients will probably benefit more from any particular approach.

Factors that may compromise hypnotic responsiveness

Apart from specific correlates of hypnotic responsiveness in childhood, such as age and hypnotisability, several variables that are not directly related to hypnotic ability may enhance or impede hypnotic responsiveness in a clinical setting. These are briefly described below.

Parents' myths and misconceptions about hypnosis

To prepare the child to learn techniques of hypnosis and self-hypnosis, the parents' expectations need to be discussed and clarified first. Usually children look to their parents for guidance and assurance when facing new situations, and if the parents communicate a confident attitude towards hypnosis, the child is much more likely to be trusting and co-operative.

Gardner[34] described techniques designed to help parents who are dubious about hypnosis to move from being obstacles to becoming allies in their children's treatment. The approach includes three basic components:

1 *educational*: eliciting and responding to parents' specific questions and concerns
2 *observational*: parents observing their children in hypnosis
3 *experiential*: parents experiencing hypnosis themselves.

Parents may be reluctant to allow their child to undergo hypnosis for a variety of reasons, generally related to something they have been told by someone else, or that they have read about in a novel or spy story, or that they may have seen on television or on stage (in countries such as the UK, where stage hypnosis is legal). Box 5.1 provides a list of the commonest misconceptions about hypnosis that are presented by parents of children with cancer.[35]

Box 5.1:   Common misconceptions about hypnosis

- The child will not be in control of him- or herself, and the therapist will be in control of him or her.
- The child will do something that they might not otherwise do.
- The child will say something that they had not meant to say.
- Only very stupid and very suggestible people can be hypnotised.
- Only dependent people can be hypnotised.
- The child may remain 'stuck' in hypnosis.
- The child will not remember what has happened in hypnosis.

It is imperative to deal with all of the most popular misconceptions held by parents about hypnosis before attempting an induction procedure with the child.

Children's misconceptions about hypnosis

In most cases, children do not have mistaken (or indeed any) notions about hypnosis. It is usually sufficient to ask the child what they know about hypnosis. In most instances, children have seen a television or film dramatisation of hypnosis. They can be told something similar to the following: 'Lots of times things are exaggerated on television. In the hospital we only use hypnosis for important things like helping children to feel better during chemotherapy and to feel in control of medical procedures'.

Staff preparation

Misconceptions, negative attitudes and a lack of information about hypnosis among health professionals limit the number of children who are referred for hypnotherapy, and they can sabotage ongoing hypnotherapy by a qualified professional with a motivated and capable child.

Case history 5.1

Peter was a 7-year-old boy with moderate to high hypnotic ability. He was well motivated to reduce his venepuncture and lumbar puncture-related pain by means of hypnosis, and he was very successful in doing so. During one of his training sessions a member of the cleaning staff entered the room unexpectedly, saw him undergoing hypnosis and commented 'What are you doing there? Only stupid people do things like that – you are a man now'. Despite the best efforts of the psychologist and his parents, Peter never tried hypnosis again. He received general anaesthesia for his subsequent lumbar punctures, and was experiencing considerable pain during his venepunctures, despite the application of a local anaesthetic throughout the rest of his treatment.

In summary, prior to conducting any form of hypnosis, it is essential to remove any misconceptions that may be held by patients, parents or staff. Hypnotherapy can be undermined by opponents of its use, and therefore it is essential to secure the co-operation of all those involved in the child's care.

Hypnotic intervention studies for paediatric procedure-related cancer pain

The experience of paediatric procedure-related cancer pain has been the focus of numerous case reports and an increasing number of systematic studies. This chapter will focus on systematic studies of hypnotic interventions that have been published since 1981. (For a comprehensive review of the relevant studies, *see* Liossi.[36])

Zeltzer and LeBaron[37] compared hypnotic and non-hypnotic behavioural techniques with regard to efficacy in reducing pain and anxiety in 33 patients aged from 6 to 17 years and with a mean time since diagnosis of 23 months. Non-hypnotic behavioural techniques included a combination of deep breathing, distraction and practice sessions to help the child to control their fear. Patients in the hypnosis group were helped to become increasingly involved in interesting and pleasant images, and were also instructed to take deep breaths and have practice sessions.

For both lumbar puncture and bone-marrow aspiration procedures, intervention was associated with an overall reduction in pain. A significant interaction that was found between the amount of pain reduction and the type of intervention suggested that hypnosis was mainly responsible for the decrease in pain, and *post-hoc* analyses confirmed this finding. Anxiety during procedures was also reduced by intervention. Although the hypnosis group showed a large decrease in anxiety, only a small reduction in anxiety was found in the non-hypnosis group.

Katz and colleagues[38] compared the effects of hypnosis with play comparison interventions in the reduction of pain and distress in 36 children with acute lymphoblastic leukaemia, aged between 6 and 12 years, undergoing repeated bone-marrow aspirations. Time since diagnosis ranged from 3 months to 6 years 5 months, with a mean of 2 years 5 months (SD = 2.13 years). Components of the hypnotic intervention included the development of rapport, direct discussions about the child's medical history and treatment needs, a hypnotic induction utilising eye fixation (with or without eye closure), active imagery tailored to the interests of each individual child, deep muscle relaxation, and suggestions. The specific suggestions that were incorporated included imagery to reduce or reframe sensory/pain experiences, distraction and relaxation, pairing positive affect with medical procedures, developing a sense of mastery and control over sensory and affective experience, and post-hypnotic suggestions for practising and re-entering hypnosis with a cue from their therapist during actual procedures. The comparison study condition consisted of non-directed play sessions that were designed to control the amount of time and attention that the child received from the psychologist who was performing the hypnotic intervention. Elements of the non-directed play condition included development of rapport, non-medical play and non-medical verbal interaction.

Children in both hypnosis and comparison groups demonstrated significant decreases in self-report of fear and pain from baseline to post-intervention bone-marrow aspirations, with no major differences between groups.

Kuttner and colleagues[39] compared behavioural/hypnotic 'imaginative involvement', and a standard medical practice control group with regard to the reduction in procedural pain and distress during bone-marrow aspiration in 30 children aged 3 to 10 years. In the distraction intervention, the child was shown toys, puppets, pop-up books, was asked distracting questions, and was engaged in physical activities such as blowing bubbles and squeezing Mum's hand. The hypnotic group received a combination of hypnotic suggestion, guided imagery and therapist support. The standard medical practice control group received information about the procedure when the child entered the treatment room and during the procedure, as well as emotional support. Following treatment, each child was assessed during two consecutive bone-marrow aspirations. The only significant finding to emerge indicated that, among younger children (age range 3 years to 6 years 11 months), the hypnotic treatment produced lower distress scores than did the distraction or control treatments in the first bone-marrow aspiration only. By the second bone-marrow aspiration, the younger children in the three groups showed equivalent decreases in distress scores. There were no significant differences in self-reported pain and anxiety between the three groups.

Wall and Womack[40] examined the differential effects of standardised instruction in hypnosis or an active cognitive strategy for provision of relief from procedure-related pain and anxiety. In the active cognitive strategy, patients were trained to use their own chosen distraction during the bone-marrow aspiration or lumbar puncture. The participants were 20 paediatric oncology outpatients ranging in age from 5 to 18 years. Interventions consisted of group practice training sessions, where each group met twice in the week in which they were to receive a bone-marrow aspiration or lumbar puncture. This study appears to be unique in its approach to the use of group-training sessions. At the time of the second bone-marrow aspiration or lumbar puncture, patients were cued by tape to make use of the techniques learned during the training sessions. The headphones were removed prior to the preparation (site cleansing) of patients for bone-marrow aspiration or lumbar puncture. The authors concluded that although both techniques appeared to be significantly effective in decreasing pain, neither was more effective than the other, and neither appeared to be effective in anxiety reduction.

Liossi and Hatira[41] conducted a controlled trial to compare the efficacy of clinical hypnosis vs. cognitive–behavioural (CB) training in alleviating the pain and distress of 30 paediatric cancer patients (aged 5 to 15 years) undergoing bone-marrow aspirations. Patients were randomised to one of three groups, namely hypnosis, a package of CB coping skills, and no intervention. In the hypnosis group, children received hypnotic analgesic suggestions (i.e. a request for numbness, topical, local and glove anaesthesia) and were given post-hypnotic suggestions. In the CB group, children were taught relaxation training, breathing exercises and cognitive restructuring. In the control group, children (like those in all groups) received a standard lidocaine injection. The results demonstrated that patients who received either hypnosis or CB reported less pain and pain-related anxiety than did control patients, and also reported less pain and anxiety than at their own baseline. Hypnosis and CB were similarly effective in relieving pain. The results also indicated that children reported more anxiety and displayed more behavioural distress in the CB group than in the hypnosis group.

Liossi and Hatira[42] also conducted a prospective controlled trial to investigate the efficacy of a manual-based clinical hypnosis intervention in alleviating the pain of 80 paediatric cancer patients (6–16 years of age) undergoing regular lumbar punctures. Patients were randomly assigned to one of four groups, namely direct hypnosis with standard medical treatment, indirect hypnosis with standard medical treatment, attention control with standard medical treatment and standard medical treatment alone. The results confirmed that patients in the hypnosis groups reported less pain and anxiety and were rated as displaying less behavioural distress than patients in the control groups. Direct and indirect suggestions were equally effective. The level of hypnotisability was significantly associated with the magnitude of treatment benefit in the hypnosis groups. For both hypnosis groups, the therapeutic benefit decreased when patients were switched to self-hypnosis. The investigators concluded that hypnosis is effective in preparing paediatric oncology patients for lumbar puncture, but that the presence of the therapist may be critical for success.

To facilitate comparison of the important elements of the studies reviewed here, Table 5.1 cites each of the studies reviewed and includes a description of the participants, the research design, the major procedures and the major findings.

The consistency of the findings reported above indicates the usefulness of hypnosis as an effective intervention for helping children and adolescents to control pain and anxiety associated with medical procedures, and it renders hypnosis an empirically validated intervention[5.1] in procedure-related pain management.

Mechanisms of hypnotic analgaesia

Investigations of potential mechanisms of hypnotic analgesia can be broadly divided into those that emphasise psychological processes and those that emphasise physiological processes. The actual mechanisms are likely to be complex, so the various psychological and physiological explanations need not be mutually exclusive.

Patterson and colleagues[44] suggest a hierarchical pain control model articulated by Kiernan *et al.*[45] as being useful in organising theory about hypnotic analgesia. The model of Kiernan *et al.*[45] neatly conceptualises the possible multiple actions of a pain control intervention, and consists of three levels:

1 spinal cord antinociceptive mechanisms
2 higher cortical mechanisms that serve to prevent awareness of pain once nociception has been transmitted
3 a selective reduction in the affective dimension of pain, as a consequence of reinterpretation of meanings associated with the painful sensation.

Research studies investigating hypnotic analgesia at a basic physiological level suggest the possibility that such analgesia involves centrifugal inhibition of nociceptive transmission. Recent physiological studies have focused primarily on autonomic,[46–48] neurochemical,[49–51] and electrocortical[52,53] changes associated with hypnotic analgesia, and these studies have provided valuable information. However, they have considerable limitations – for example, it is difficult to identify precisely the general neuroanatomical sites at which the relevant modulatory

---

5.1 According to Chambless and Hollon,[43] for a treatment to be considered *efficacious* for a particular population there must be at least two different between-group design experiments, conducted by at least two different research teams, demonstrating that the intervention in question is superior to a non-treatment control condition, an alternative treatment or a placebo, or that the treatment is equivalent to a previously established efficacious treatment. To be designated *possibly efficacious* for a particular population, there need only be one between-group design study of a treatment that meets these criteria. Finally, to be considered *efficacious and specific*, a treatment must be shown by two different teams to be superior to a placebo or to a treatment of previously established efficacy in studies that control for non-specific processes. To ensure valid treatment implementation, studies must utilise treatment manuals, except where the treatment is simple and adequately described in the journal article.

Table 5.1: Hypnotic intervention studies for paediatric procedure-related cancer pain

Study	Patients (n)	Age range (years)	Design	Interventions	Outcome measures	Results
Zeltzer and LeBaron	33	6–17	Repeated measures, factorial	Hypnosis: therapist-assisted imagery Non-hypnotic condition: deep breathing, distraction (counting, hand squeezing and talking)	Self-reported pain, self-reported anxiety	Bone-marrow aspirations: pain specifically reduced in both treatment groups, anxiety reduced in hypnosis/imagery group only Lumbar puncture: pain significantly reduced in hypnosis/imagery group only, anxiety significantly reduced in both treatment groups Overall hypnosis/imagery associated with greater reduction in pain and anxiety than distraction
Katz et al.	36	6–12	Repeated measures, factorial	Hypnosis: (induction) eye fixation with or without eye closure, imagery, muscle relaxation, and suggestion related to coping with sensory aspects of bone-marrow aspiration Post-hypnotic suggestion for re-entering hypnosis with cue from therapist Control: unstructured play sessions prior to bone-marrow aspiration	PBRS-r, nurse rating of anxiety, self-reported fear, self-reported pain, therapist–patient rapport ratings, and response to hypnosis ratings	No significant difference in distress between groups, distress scores increased from first to third bone-marrow aspiration, equivalent reductions in self-reported pain and fear from baseline to post-treatment in both groups, consistent increase in scores from first to second bone-marrow aspiration

Table 5.1: Continued

Study	Patients (n)	Age range (years)	Design	Interventions	Outcome measures	Results
Kuttner et al.	30	3–10	Repeated measures, factorial	Distraction: bubble blowing, pop-up books, puppet play, deep breathing Hypnotic 'imaginative involvement': suggestions for time reduction, analgesia using a pain switch technique, and imaginary stories Control: standard practice	Self-reported pain, self-reported anxiety, PBRS-r, observer-rated pain, observer-rated anxiety	No significant difference in distress scores for older children; younger children in hypnosis groups had lower distress scores on first bone-marrow aspiration only, no significant difference in pain and anxiety among groups
Wall and Womack	20	5–18	Repeated measures, factorial	Hypnosis: (induction) arm levitation, relaxation, visual imagery, cued to use hypnosis with taped message Active cognitive strategy: procedural information plus distraction activities	Self-reported anxiety, self-reported pain, observer-rated pain and observer-rated anxiety	Both interventions were effective in reducing pain but not anxiety No difference in pain or anxiety reduction between groups
Liossi and Hatira	30	5–15	Parallel group	Hypnosis: (induction) relaxation and visual imagery, request for numbness, topical, local and glove anaesthesia Cognitive–behavioural training: relaxation, breathing exercises, and cognitive restructuring Control: lidocaine	Self-reported pain, self-reported anxiety and PBCL	Hypnosis and cognitive-behavioural training were equally effective in the relief of pain Children reported more anxiety and exhibited more behavioural distress in the cognitive–behavioural training condition

| Liossi and Hatira | 80 | 6–16 | Parallel group | Hypnosis direct: request for numbness, topical, local and glove anaesthesia, switchbox Hypnosis indirect: metaphors Attention control Control: standard practice | Self-reported pain, self-reported anxiety and PBCL | Hypnosis was effective in the relief of pain, anxiety and behavioural distress |

PBRS-r, Procedural Behavior Rating Scale – Revised; PBCL, Procedure Behavior Check List.

mechanisms operate.[45] Moreover, the results of most of these studies are subject to multiple interpretations and leave many unanswered questions about possible antinociceptive mechanisms.[54–56]

Kiernan et al.[45] investigated the mechanisms of hypnotic analgesia by measuring changes in the R-III,[5.2] a nociceptive spinal reflex, during hypnotic reduction of pain sensation and unpleasantness. The R-III was measured in 15 healthy volunteers who gave Visual Analogue Scale (VAS) sensory and affective ratings of an electrical stimulus during conditions of resting wakefulness, hypnotic analgesic suggestions, and deliberate attempted suppression of the reflex during non-hypnotic conditions. The H-reflex was also measured to control for general changes in alpha-motoneurone excitability. The results showed that both hypnotic sensory analgesia and hypnotic affective analgesia were related to a decrease in the R-III. The latter was 67% as great and accounted for 51% of the variance in the decrease in pain sensation. In turn, the reduction in pain sensation was 75% as great and accounted for 77% of the variance in the decrease in unpleasantness. Hypnotic suggestions for sensory analgesia were not more effective in reducing pain sensation or unpleasantness of the R-III than were hypnotic suggestions for comfort and well-being. A moderate correlation was found between hypnotisability and sensory analgesia (tau B $= 0.45$; $P < 0.01$), but no significant correlations were found between susceptibility and affective analgesia (tau B $= 0.27$; $P = 0.08$) or between susceptibility and hypnotic reduction of R-III (tau B $= 0.27$; $P = 0.1$). It is important to note that hypnotic suggestion resulted in a reduction in R-III which was only 67% as large as the reduction in pain sensation. This is in contrast to similarly designed studies of morphine analgesia which showed that the latter reduces pain intensity and R-III on a nearly equal percentage basis.[57]

The next level of hypnotic pain control discussed by Kiernan et al.[45] is related to the ability of higher cortical functions to keep incoming nociceptive signals out of conscious awareness. This level of control is described in different ways by a variety of psychological theories, the most prominent being the neodissociation[54] and sociocognitive[58] theories. According to the neodissociation theory, hypnotic analgesia produces reduced awareness of pain by generating an amnesia-like barrier after nociceptive information has reached the higher centres.[59] According to the sociocognitive theory, social demand characteristics and the possible role of deception cannot be ignored in the interpretation of hypnotic analgesia.[60] Laboratory-based studies suggest that individuals with a wide range of hypnotisability are capable of this level of

---

5.2   The R-III is a spinally mediated nociceptive reflex that is maintained after transection of the spinal cord. Its latency is consistent with the conduction velocity of group III (Aδ) afferents, and its magnitude is related to subjective pain intensity.

pain control,[54,58] that patient expectations and contextual factors play a significant role in determining success,[58] and that responsiveness to hypnosis can be enhanced by means of various experiential and training procedures.[58]

The final level of hypnotic pain control proposed by Kiernan *et al.*[45] is related to the affective dimension of pain. Sensory pain is thought to be linked more directly to nociceptive input, whereas affective responses are more under the control of higher cognitive interpretation of pain sensations. As such, the affective dimension of pain is more influenced by the perceived context of the pain.[59] Furthermore, affective responses can presumably be influenced more by the process of reinterpretation, such as suggestions to experience the situation as being more pleasant. Laboratory research suggests that individuals are able to achieve greater reductions in the affective vs. sensory dimension of painful stimuli with hypnosis.[31] Direct suggestion without hypnotic induction has also been found to decrease the affective dimension of pain in the laboratory.[61] The positive effects of suggestions on the affective pain dimension have been found to be unrelated to hypnotic responsivity.[31] Because hypnosis affects pain and suffering at a very high level of neural organisation – consciousness itself – its effect is apparently not a function of the source or type of pain involved. Any pain, whether it is peripheral or central, lancinating or dull, burning or cold, resulting from injury or disease, benign or malignant, acute or chronic, can be reinterpreted by consciousness so that it is no longer painful or a cause of suffering.

Description of hypnotic techniques

Physical surroundings

Ideally, the technique should be taught in a quiet area, uninterrupted, with the telephone diverted and the patient lying in bed. Although a quiet environment is always preferable during the training sessions, in hospital settings interruptions are frequent. If these are incorporated into the induction and imagery, the patient can continue to remain deeply relaxed. For example, we can say to the patient something like: 'And just allow any sounds to drift away, reminding you that it is possible to be so comfortable and far away that it really doesn't matter'.

The overall plan of the hypnotic interventions

The process of clinical hypnosis can be divided conceptually into six phases as follows:[62]

1 preparation
2 induction
3 deepening
4 therapeutic suggestions
5 post-hypnotic suggestions
6 termination.

The hypnotist develops an overall plan of the hypnotic session by choosing tasks for each phase and arranging specific suggestions accordingly. As a general rule, we start with the simplest and most direct strategies and move on to more complex ones depending on the patient's response. The specific strategies and combinations of strategies that are selected are based on our case formulation and treatment goals.

The pre-induction interview

Depending on the needs of the child, the pre-induction interview can be quite brief or more extensive. The interview includes discussion of the reasons for utilising hypnosis, clarification of misconceptions, and a full response to questions. Details of the child's likes and dislikes, significant experiences, fears, hopes and comfort areas are discussed. It is essential that the child forms a comfortable, trusting relationship with the therapist and feels safe with him or her.[27] Hypnotic treatment does not require passive submission, but instead emphasises the child's involvement and control of the situation, and allows the child to participate actively and enthusiastically in his or her own treatment.

Hypnotic induction techniques for children

Hilgard and LeBaron[63] describe induction procedures as simple procedures 'designed to provide a gradual transition from our usual generalised reality orientation to the limited orientation characteristic of hypnosis'. Children respond to a considerable number of hypnotic induction techniques, each of which has many variations. Most include instructing the individual to focus attention, to attend to the hypnotist, to relax, and eventually to close the eyes and follow what the hypnotist is suggesting. Any induction method may also be used as a deepening method, and methods may be combined. The choice of an appropriate induction for any particular child will depend on the needs and preferences of the child and the skills and training of the therapist.

Compared with adults, children are more likely to fidget and move about, open their eyes, or refuse to close them, and make spontaneous comments during hypnosis. Many children have negative attitudes to going to sleep, and therefore words such as 'sleepy' should be avoided in the inductions. Similarly, since some young children resist closing their eyes, eye closure should not be stressed as imperative to induction. The language should be adapted to the child's developmental level, neither talking down to them nor using overly complex terms. Positive feedback to the child's responses should be given, and expectations of success should be communicated by focusing on possibilities and avoiding words such as 'try' which imply that failure may be the outcome.[27]

Olness and Gardner[27] have divided induction techniques into visual imagery, auditory imagery, movement imagery, story-telling techniques, ideomotor techniques, progressive relaxation, eye fixation, distraction, and utilisation (the use of videotapes and audiotapes or of the telephone).

Children of different ages often prefer different induction techniques. Although techniques can be grouped according to the age groups for which they are most appropriate (*see* Box 5.2), their appropriateness varies, especially in cases where levels of cognitive or social–emotional development deviate from expectations based on chronological age.[27] The choice of an appropriate induction technique depends on the needs and preferences of the child, as well as on the experience, creativity and preferences of the therapist.

The descriptions of techniques that follow consist of the actual words that can be said to a child. Obviously the phrasing will vary from one

---

Box 5.2:   Hypnotic induction techniques categorised by age group

3–6 years
Favourite place
Story-telling
Television fantasy

7–11 years
Favourite place
Favourite activity
Arm rigidity

12–16 years
Favourite place
Sports activity
Arm rigidity
Playing music
Indirect (Ericksonian) techniques

child to another, and from one time to another. It is emphasised that these are merely samples, and that variations are both necessary and appropriate in actual clinical practice.

Visual imagery

Favourite place

> As you are feeling more relaxed, just allow your mind to go to a very special place – a place where you feel peaceful, tranquil and safe. It may be a new place, one that you have never been to before, or it may be a place you have been to before. What is important is that you go to this special place and begin to notice what is around you.

We then make suggestions to facilitate the deepening of this experience. These include noticing all the surrounding details – seeing shapes, colour and light, hearing sounds, feeling the air and sun against one's face, smelling whatever is in the air, and touching things nearby.

> It might be easier if you close your eyes, but you can leave them open if you like, or leave them open until you close them.

If the child cannot think of a place we can suggest something like the following:

> Now I want you to imagine that it is a very, very warm summer evening, and you are lying on a beach in . . . . You can feel a warm breeze flow across your body and through your hair. And you can smell the salty air of the sea. The sky and the sea are a perfectly clear blue . . . and the sun is just about to set. It's a beautiful, burnt-orange colour. And you can feel the warmth of the sun pouring into every muscle of your body. In the distance, you can hear the seagulls . . . and you can see the waves as they roll in and they roll back out again. You can see a sailing boat on the horizon. You can feel the warmth of the sand beneath you . . . and you can hear the waves as they roll in, and roll back out again . . . roll in, and roll back out again . . . . Take some time to enjoy it. When you feel as if you are really there, let me know by lifting one finger to say yes.

Favourite activity

> Tell me something you like to do. (The child answers.) Good. Just imagine that you can see yourself doing that. Let yourself really enjoy it.

Television (or film) fantasy[27]

> You told me you like to watch TV and that your favourite pro-gramme is . . . . Just imagine yourself getting ready to watch your favourite TV programme. Where is the TV set you are watching? Just get comfortable, and when you are ready turn to the channel you want. Now you can see your favourite programme. Adjust the sound and the picture and when they are just right for you, let me know by lifting one finger. Good. Just continue watching and listen-ing, feeling very comfortable, very good.

Auditory imagery[27]

Playing a musical instrument

> You said that you like to play the guitar. When and where do you like to do that best? Good. Imagine that you are there now, playing your favourite piece. Listen through the piece in your mind. Enjoy playing it very well, making just the sounds that you like. When you have come to the end of the piece, let me know by lifting one finger.

The patient can be asked to tap out the beat with their foot. When the tapping ceases, the therapist will know that the patient has finished the piece.

Movement imagery[27]

Sports activity

> You told me you like to do fencing . . . . Imagine yourself fencing, wearing your white uniform, your colourful glove, rattling your foil and scoring points against your opponent . . . . Let yourself get very comfortable as you imagine a game. Feel your control as your muscles and foil move the way you tell them – running, jump-ing, attacking your opponent or defending yourself. Enjoy being with the winning team and continue until the game is won and you are given a medal. Let me know when the game is over by lifting one finger.

Story-telling techniques[27]

With young children or those who are too anxious to participate in other imagery techniques, the therapist can make up a story suited to the child's needs and interests. The story can be an entirely new fantasy production or a variation of a TV programme or a fairy tale or other theme with which the child is familiar. The therapist either takes full responsibility for the story or asks the child to contribute ideas to the extent that they are able and willing to do so.

Ideomotor techniques

Ideomotor techniques involve asking the child to focus mentally on the idea of a particular movement and to let the movement occur without conscious muscle activity. The most commonly used ideomotor techniques, namely those of arm lowering, arm levitation and arm rigidity, are described below.

Arm lowering

We will count from 1 to 3. One, look up with your eyes as far as you can without moving your head. Up, up, that's right. Two, slowly close your eyelids, keep your eyes up, while you take a deep breath. Good. Three, as you let the breath out, let your eyes relax and let your body feel twice as relaxed. Fine. Now I will raise your hand. (Hold the hand about a foot off the lap.) Let your hand feel very heavy, as if heavy books are attached to it. That's right, very heavy. (Wait until the arm and hand loosen and relax. Give more suggestion if needed.) Very heavy, as if it is just too much trouble to hold it up, as if all of your schoolbooks are on it. Now, as your arm drops to your lap, you can feel twice as relaxed as before, deeply comfortable and relaxed.

Hand levitation

Perhaps you'd like just to sit comfortably in the chair and let your hands rest lightly on your thighs. You may close your eyes. Notice the feelings and sensations in your hands and in your fingers. You can feel the texture of the cloth, the warmth of your thighs, perhaps a little tingling sensation in your fingers or in the palms of your hands. You may be interested in noticing the beginning of a feeling of motion in one of your fingers . . . that sensation becoming stronger and stronger. . . . It's now beginning to lift. Now feel the lightness of the finger next to it, now the next one, and feel the entire hand now lifting, higher and higher. And as that hand lifts higher and higher, notice that a feeling of comfort and relaxation continues, and spreads all over your body.

Arm rigidity

Stretch one arm straight out to the side and make a tight fist. Imagine that the arm is very strong, as if it is made of steel. Stronger and stronger. So strong that I cannot push it down. I cannot bend it. That arm is very powerful. It can be as strong and powerful as it wants.

Deepening techniques

The staircase technique

The therapist can say to the patient:

Perhaps you would like to imagine that you are at the top of a beautiful staircase and I am standing right next to you. The staircase is covered by a rich, luxurious carpet. Notice what colour the carpet is and describe it to me. (Patient responds.) That's right, it is red . . . . You are standing with bare feet on the carpet. As you stand there, you can feel your feet sink into the soft richness of this warm red carpet. As you go down the stairs, I will go down with you, step by step, and I will count the steps. As you go further and further down, you will be more and more deeply relaxed. Now let's step down to the second step. Soon you will reach the bottom of the staircase. . . . At the bottom of the staircase . . . 8 . . . 9 . . . closer and closer to the bottom of the staircase . . . 10! You are feeling so comfortable there.

The elevator and escalator techniques

Variations of the staircase technique are elevator and escalator techniques. In the elevator technique it is suggested to the patient that they are inside an elevator that can take them down deeper and deeper (or up higher and higher) in hypnosis. They could see the numbers of the floors light up above the elevator door, going from 20 to 1 or from 1 to 20. Depending on whether the patient likes to have control or likes to have things happen to them, they may or may not be told that they have the control of the elevator in their hand.

In the escalator technique, the patient is told that they are going to step on to an escalator that will transport them smoothly into hypnosis or to their favourite place. The hypnotist may suggest that the patient has the control stick for the escalator in their hand. If they pull the stick close to themselves very fast, they will go into hypnosis fast. If they pull it slowly, they will go into hypnosis slowly.

With all induction and deepening techniques, the therapist should talk to the patient in a gentle, calm, rhythmical manner. Usually the patient's breathing will slow down as they go into hypnosis. The therapist should link the rhythm of their speech to that of the patient's breathing.

Analgesic suggestions

Once patients have enjoyed being relaxed, we bring in analgesic suggestions (summarised in Box 5.3) which have been developed during the pain assessment phase.

Pain displacement

This technique involves imagining a similar or different sensation in a different part of one's body where it is less painful or distressing. Because moving pain is sometimes easier than eliminating it, pain displacement can be a valuable technique that can serve to increase the confidence of young patients. A useful suggestion for creating displacement is as follows:

Box 5.3:   Hypnotic suggestions for procedure-related pain control

Direct suggestions
Glove anaesthesia
Topical anaesthesia
Local anaesthesia
Switchbox
Pain displacement
Symptom substitution
Time distortion
Pain relief imagery

Indirect suggestions
Therapeutic stories and metaphors
Interspersal

You may already have noticed that the pain moves, ever so slightly . . . . As you continue to attend to that movement, you may notice that the pain has somehow moved out of your lower back and seems to be staying in your left hand.

Symptom substitution

Symptom substitution involves imagining substituting something else for the pain, which is similar but that hurts much less or is less intense. For example, a burning pain might be transformed by the imagination into an itch.

Time distortion

With this technique, the therapist suggests that time spent in pain is speeding up compared with normal time.

Request for numbness

We'll do some strong magic now . . . first you have to allow your back to go to sleep for a few minutes. . . . I'll show you how to do it . . . I'll just put my hand up on your back to help it become numb . . . sleepy and numb . . . soft and sleepy.

Topical anaesthesia

Just imagine painting numbing medicine on to your back.

Local anaesthesia

Imagine injecting an anaesthetic into your lower back . . . feel it flow into your body . . . notice the change in feeling as the area becomes numb.

Glove anaesthesia

Pay attention to your hand . . . notice how you can feel tingling feelings in that hand ... let it become numb . . . when it is very numb, touch that hand to your lower back . . . let the numb feeling transfer from your hand to your back.

Switchbox

The therapist explains to the child the idea that pain is transmitted by nerves from various parts of the body to the brain, which then sends a 'pain message' back to the body (coloured drawings can be used to facilitate this explanation). The patient is asked to choose a switch that can turn off or modulate incoming nerve signals situated wherever they want (e.g. in the brain or near the site of pain). Patients are asked to practise turning off the switches for defined periods of time, starting with 10–15 seconds and working up to longer periods.

Dissociation

Sensory hypnotic suggestions can also create dissociation from pain. In such cases, the patient is able to describe the pain accurately, but with a sense of distance and with no affective involvement. That is, the pain is still perceived but the patient no longer suffers from it.

A suggestion for creating dissociation might begin as follows:

It is unnecessary for you to have to stay here in the treatment room, conscious of all the routine that occurs. I wonder if you might prefer to enjoy a kind of holiday from this room. You might like to imagine you are stepping out of the room, walking down the corridor and settling nicely into the playroom. Or you might prefer to feel as if you are enjoying a lovely sunny afternoon playing ball on the beach and swimming in the cool sea. Your body can remain here in the treatment room, in order that the necessary procedure is administered, but your mind can take you far away, and you can enjoy whatever you'd like, with nothing to bother you, with no need to be aware of the treatment room or the hospital.

Indirect hypnotic suggestions

Out of his experience with hypnosis, Milton Erickson devised new, innovative methods that are very different from conventional hypnosis. In Ericksonian hypnosis, the hypnotist is informal and conversational. He/she employs indirect communication to activate a process of unconscious search within the patient. The communications are non-specific, indirect, ambiguous and often disguised. Suggestions may be embedded within ordinary conversation. Certain key phrases may be embedded or implicit in anecdotes, stories, analogies, metaphors, juxtaposition of opposites, puns, jokes and binds. These devices are intended to disrupt the patient's habitual frames of reference and to invite the patient to search for new response possibilities. Below are two therapeutic metaphors that have been found effective in the treatment of procedure-related cancer pain.

The setting sun metaphor (adapted from Levitan[64]):

> See yourself sitting on a beautiful beach at sunset. . . . Notice the bright red sun as it descends on the far horizon . . . see the sun gradually sink into the sea . . . . See the colours change from red to purple and then to blue. . . . Enjoy the tranquillity . . . tranquillity is available to you whenever you need it, merely by giving yourself your own personal signal to relax!

Mexican food metaphor (adapted from Hammond[65]):

> I remember the first time that I ever ate Mexican food. . . . I ate meat balls with red pepper in New Mexico. It contained so much red pepper that my nose started running, my eyes watered and my mouth kept burning no matter how much cold water I drank . . . but I spent the next year living in New Mexico. . . . I don't know how or when, but my body changed and adapted . . . or perhaps it was my mind that changed . . . my mouth adapted . . . almost as if, somehow, my mouth had developed a callus.

Post-hypnotic suggestions

A post-hypnotic suggestion is a suggestion that is intended to have an effect after hypnosis has ended. In general, post-hypnotic suggestions include a cue that initiates the suggested experience (or behaviour). Once the patient is in hypnosis, post-hypnotic suggestions are built into the imagery. We suggest that patients take both a visual and a 'feeling' picture of just how they are now. At any time when they would like to recapture this feeling of comfort, they need only take a deep, slow breath and take out their mental picture and they will once again feel their bodies relax as the tension flows out and comfort flows in. And whenever they need it, they can bring in the analgesic image and suggestions and increase their comfort even more.

Termination

When choosing a method of terminating hypnosis, the therapist should take into account the patient's need for structure. Compared with adults, children usually need less formality and ritual. If structure seems to be helpful, the therapist can count or ask the patient to count to a certain number, using suggestions that they will open their eyes at some point in the counting, and that they will feel fully alert, aware and refreshed by the end of the counting. If a less structured approach seems to be appropriate, the therapist can say 'Enjoy the hypnotic experience a little while longer and when you are ready, slowly, comfortably, easily, open your eyes and return to your usual state of awareness'.[27]

Self-hypnosis

The therapist teaches the patient self-hypnosis as a way to participate actively in their treatment process, to reinforce self-mastery and to promote independence. Gardner[66] described a three-step method for teaching children self-hypnosis, which can be easily accomplished in one session.

- *Step 1.* The therapist uses various induction and deepening methods, usually emphasising imagery and ideomotor techniques. After allowing time for enjoyment of the imagery, the therapist asks the child to count silently backwards from five to one, with the eyes opening at three, and fully alert at one. The therapist then comments that the child now knows how to come out of hypnosis without help. Rapid dehypnotisation in emergencies may also be discussed.
- *Step 2.* The therapist and child discuss which of the induction techniques employed in step 1 were most helpful, and agree to discard the rest. The child is then asked to describe to the therapist in detail the techniques chosen for induction, to feel the same good feelings, and to go into hypnosis easily and naturally as the description proceeds. The therapist may add details if the child's wording is too general. After another pause and a reassuring comment, the therapist then asks the child to return to the normal alert state. Problems are discussed as necessary.
- *Step 3.* This is the same as step 2, except that the child is asked to recall and to decide to experience the induction silently. Neither the child nor the therapist speaks. The child nods when hypnosis is achieved. After another pause, the child returns again to the previous alert state. Any remaining problems or questions are discussed, and the child is then ready for full independent use of self-hypnosis.

Potential adverse effects of hypnosis

Although the problem is not frequently discussed, some patients experience increased tension and anxiety during hypnosis. There are a number of measures that a therapist should take in this situation. It is of paramount importance to remain calm and to reassure the patient (verbally and non-verbally) that very soon they will feel normal again. Novice therapists in particular often pick up on the intense affect of their patients and contribute to it with their own fears and concerns. In all situations, even if the therapist is extremely concerned and anxious, they should remain calm, speak in a slow and low-pitched voice with a relaxed tone, and act as if things are going to be fine. In rare instances, traumatic material such as sexual abuse will surface spontaneously. This needs to be discussed and worked through, at least to the point at which the patient feels in control of his or her emotions. Working through intense emotional material is an important process that can be done through hypnosis, but obviously it requires a therapist who has been trained in psychotherapy.

Case history 5.2

Joanna was a 16-year-old girl with non-Hodgkin's lymphoma 6 months after the initial diagnosis. She was becoming increasingly uncomfortable and distressed about the various treatments she was receiving, and she was protesting vigorously during all painful procedures, including venepunctures. She was referred for psychological assessment and support, and from the very first sessions it became evident that she was a very bright, artistic individual who was well aware of her diagnosis, prognosis and the implications of the disease for her life. She jointly decided with the psychologist that she would like to be able to undergo all of the painful procedures without feeling extreme pain but also without having to depend on general anaesthesia. She believed that this achievement would make her feel good in herself again, give her back some control over her life, and help her to feel stronger in her battle against her disease. She had moderate to high hypnotic ability and was well motivated and keen to try everything. She was taught hypnosis and self-hypnosis, and after four 30-minute sessions she was able to undergo invasive medical procedures with minimal distress. As an induction technique she was using the arm levitation, and then she was imagining the following story.

A polar bear called Joanna decided to leave her igloo and go fishing and swimming at the nearby beach. She put on her new shiny green swimsuit and her Gucci sunglasses, then she took her fishing stick with her and set off. When she arrived at the beach she decided to do a little fishing first, so she sat down and prepared her fishing stick. She threw it backwards behind her back in order to gain momentum and reach deeper in the sea, but then an accident happened. As she was throwing it, the hook stabbed her and became stuck in her back. This was painful, but Joanna was brave and immediately reached her arm back and took the hook off her back.[5.3] After that incident she thought she had better take a relaxing swim in the cool sea. She swam a lot and after she had cooled her back enough and was feeling refreshed, she got out of the sea, lay under a palm tree and dried herself, enjoying the warm sun on her body. She wanted to get a suntan, but not too much, as she wanted to remain a polar bear and not become a brown bear! After that she met up with her friends who had gone sailing, and they all had lunch – salmon caught by her friends.

References

1   Esdaile J (1957) *Hypnosis in Medicine and Surgery*. Julian, New York.

2   Hilgard ER and Hilgard JR (1994) *Hypnosis in the Relief of Pain*. Brunner/Mazel, New York.

3   Liossi C (2000) Clinical hypnosis in pediatric oncology: a critical review of the literature. *Sleep and Hypnosis*. **1**: 268–74.

4   American Psychological Association (1994) APA definition and description of hypnosis. Defining hypnosis for the public. *Contemp Hypnosis*. **11**: 142–3.

5   Bowers KS (1966) Hypnotic behavior: the differentiation of trance and demand characteristic variables. *J Abnorm Psychol*. **71**: 42–51.

6   Orne MT (1959) The nature of hypnosis: artifact and essence. *J Abnorm Psychol*. **58**: 277–99.

7   Sarbin TR (1950) Contributions to role-taking theory. I. Hypnotic behavior. *Psychol Rev*. **57**: 225–70.

8   Barber TX (1969) *Hypnosis: a scientific approach*. Van Nostrand Reinhold, New York.

9   Kirsch I and Lynn SJ (1995) The altered state of hypnosis. Changes in the theoretical landscape. *Am Psychol*. **50**: 846–58.

5.3   There were many variations of Joanna's accident. One day as she was swimming she stepped on an urchin that got stuck in her foot. Another day she was chased by a shark which managed to bite her back before she grabbed it and threw it on the beach, where she would eat it as her lunch later with her friends.

10 Fromm E (1992) An ego-psychological theory of hypnosis. In: E Fromm and M Nash (eds) *Contemporary Hypnosis Research*. Guilford Press, New York, 131–48.

11 Nash MR (1991) Hypnosis as a special case of psychological regression. In: SJ Lynn and JW Rhue (eds) *Theories of Hypnosis: current models and perspectives*. Guilford Press, New York, 171–94.

12 Hilgard ER (1969) Altered states of awareness. *J Nerv Ment Dis*. **149**: 68–79.

13 Kihlstom JF (1985) Hypnosis. *Annu Rev Psychol*. **36**: 385–418.

14 McConkey KM (1991) The construction and resolution of experience and behavior in hypnosis. In: SJ Lynn and JW Rhue (eds) *Theories of Hypnosis: current models and perspectives*. Guilford Press, New York, 542–63.

15 Sheehan PW (1991) Hypnosis, context and commitment. In: SJ Lynn and W Rhue (eds) *Theories of Hypnosis: current models and perspectives*. Guilford Press, New York, 540–41.

16 Coe WC and Sarbin TR (1991) Role theory: hypnosis from a dramaturgical and narrational perspective. In: SJ Lynn and JW Rhue (eds) *Theories of Hypnosis: current models and perspectives*. Guilford Press, New York, 303–23.

17 Dixon M and Laurence J (1992) Two hundred years of hypnosis research: Questions resolved? Questions unanswered! In: E Fromm and M Nash (eds) *Contemporary Hypnosis Research*. Guilford Press, New York, 34–66.

18 Kirsch I (1991) The social learning theory of hypnosis. In: SJ Lynn and J Rhue (eds) *Theories of Hypnosis: current models and perspectives*. Guilford Press, New York, 439–66.

19 Kirsch I and Council JR (1989) Response expectancy as a determinant of hypnotic behaviour. In: NP Spanos and JF Chaves (eds) *Hypnosis: the cognitive–behavioral perspective*. Prometheus Press, Buffalo, NY, 360–79.

20 Lynn SJ and Rhue JW (1991) An integrative model of hypnosis. In: SJ Lynne and JW Rhue (eds) *Theories of Hypnosis: current models and perspectives*. Guilford Press, New York, 397–438.

21 Nadon R, Laurence JR and Perry C (1991) The two disciplines of scientific hypnosis: a synergistic model. In: SJ Lynn and W Rhue (eds) *Theories of Hypnosis: current models and perspectives*. Guilford Press, New York, 485–519.

22 Spanos NP (1986) Hypnotic behavior: a social–psychological interpretation of amnesia, analgesia and 'trance logic'. *Behav Brain Sci*. **9**: 499–502.

23 Spanos NP (1991) A sociocognitive approach to hypnosis. In: SJ Lynn and JW Rhue (eds) *Theories of Hypnosis: current models and perspectives*. Guilford Press, New York, 324–61.

24 Lynn SJ and Rhue JW (eds) (1991) *Theories of Hypnosis: current models and perspectives*. Guilford Press, New York.

25 Barber T and Calverley D (1963) 'Hypnotic-like' suggestibility in children and adults. *J Abnorm Soc Psychol.* **66**: 589–97.

26 Morgan AH and Hilgard ER (1973) Age differences in susceptibility to hypnosis. *Int J Clin Exp Hypnosis.* **21**: 65–78.

27 Olness K and Gardner GG (1988) *Hypnosis and Hypnotherapy with Children* (2e). Grune and Stratton, Philadelphia, PA.

28 Hilgard E (1965) *The Experience of Hypnosis*. Harcourt Brace Jovanovich, New York.

29 Spanos NP (1989) Experimental research on hypnotic analgesia. In: NP Spanos and JF Chaves (eds) *Hypnosis: the cognitive–behavioral perspective*. Prometheus, Buffalo, NY, 206–40.

30 Spanos NP, Perlini AH and Robertson LA (1989) Hypnosis, suggestion and placebo in the reduction of experimental pain. *J Abnorm Psychol.* **98**: 285–93.

31 Price DD and Barber J (1987) A quantitative analysis of factors that contribute to the efficacy of hypnotic analgesia. *J Abnorm Psychol.* **96**: 46–51.

32 Barber J and Adrian C (eds) (1982) *Psychological Approaches to the Management of Pain*. Brunner/Mazel, New York.

33 Spiegel H and Spiegel D (1978) *Trance and Treatment: clinical uses of hypnosis*. Basic Books Inc, New York.

34 Gardner GG (1974) Parents: obstacles or allies in child hypnotherapy? *Am J Clin Hypnosis.* **17**: 44–9.

35 Liossi C (2002) Popular misconceptions regarding hypnosis among parents of children with cancer. *Contemp Hypnosis.* In press.

36 Liossi C (1999) Management of paediatric procedure-related cancer pain. *Pain Rev.* **6**: 279–302.

37 Zeltzer L and LeBaron S (1982) Hypnosis and nonhypnotic techniques for the reduction of pain and anxiety during painful procedures in children and adolescents with cancer. *J Pediatrics.* **101**: 1032–5.

38 Katz E, Kellerman J and Ellenberg L (1987) Hypnosis in the reduction of acute pain and distress in children with cancer. *J Pediatr Psychol.* **12**: 379–94.

39 Kuttner L, Bowman M and Teasdale M (1988) Psychological treatment of distress, pain and anxiety for young children with cancer. *Dev Behav Pediatrics.* **9**: 374–81.

40 Wall V and Womack W (1989) Hypnotic versus active cognitive strategies for alleviation of procedural distress in pediatric oncology patients. *Am J Clin Hypnosis.* **31**: 181–91.

41 Liossi C and Hatira P (1999) Clinical hypnosis versus cognitive behavioral training for pain management with paediatric cancer patients undergoing bone-marrow aspirations. *Int J Clin Exp Hypnosis*. **47**: 104–16.

42 Liossi C and Hatira P (2002) Clinical hypnosis in the alleviation of procedure-related pain in pediatric oncology patients. *Int J Clin Exp Hypnosis*. In press.

43 Chambless DL and Hollon SD (1998) Defining empirically supported therapies. *J Consult Clin Psychol*. **66**: 7–18.

44 Patterson DR, Adcock RJ and Bombardier CH (1997) Factors predicting hypnotic analgesia in clinical burn pain. *Int J Clin Exp Hypnosis*. **45**: 377–95.

45 Kiernan BD, Dane JR, Phillips LH and Price DD (1995) Hypnotic analgesia reduces R-III nociceptive reflex: further evidence concerning the multifactorial nature of hypnotic analgesia. *Pain*. **60**: 39–47.

46 Evans M and Paul G (1970) Effects of hypnotically suggested analgesia on physiological and subjective responses to cold stress. *J Consult Clin Psychol*. **35**: 362–71.

47 Hilgard ER, Morgan AH, Lange AF *et al*. (1974) Heart rate changes in pain and hypnosis. *Psychophysiology*. **11**: 692–702.

48 Sarbin TR and Slagle RW (1979) Hypnosis and psychophysiological outcomes. In: E Fromm and RE Shor (eds) *Hypnosis: developments in research and new perspectives*. Aldine, New York, 273–303.

49 Goldstein A and Hilgard ER (1975) Lack of influence of the morphine antagonist naloxone on hypnotic analgesia. *Proc Natl Acad Sci*. **72**: 2041–3.

50 Mayer DJ, Price DD, Barber J and Rajii A (1976) Acupuncture analgesia: evidence for activation of a pain-inhibitory system as a mechanism of action. In: JJ Bonica and D Albe-Fessard (eds) *Advances of Pain Research and Therapy. Vol. 1*. Raven, New York, 751–4.

51 Barber J and Mayer D (1977) Evaluation of the efficacy and neural mechanism of a hypnotic analgesia procedure in experimental and clinical dental pain. *Pain*. **4**: 41–8.

52 Karlin R, Morgan D and Goldstein L (1980) Hypnotic analgesia: a preliminary investigation of quantitated hemispheric electroencephalographic and attentional correlates. *J Abnorm Psychol*. **89**: 591–4.

53 Crawford HJ and Gruzelier JH (1992) A midstream view of the neuropsychology of hypnosis: recent research and future directions. In: E Fromm and MR Nash (eds) *Contemporary Hypnosis Research*. Guilford Press, New York.

54 Hilgard ER (1973) A neodissociation interpretation of pain reduction in hypnosis. *Psychol. Rev*. **80**: 396–411.

55   DeBenedittis G, Panerai AA and Villamira MA (1989) Effects of hypnotic analgesia and hypnotisability on experimental ischemic pain. *Int J Clin Exp Hypnosis*. **37**: 55–69.

56   Zachariae R and Bjerring P (1990) The effect of hypnotically induced analgesia on flare reaction of cutaneous histamine prick test. *Arch Dermatol Res*. **282**: 539–43.

57   Willer JC (1985) Studies on pain. Effects of morphine on a spinal nociceptive flexion reflex and related pain sensation in man. *Brain Res*. **331**: 105–14.

58   Chaves JF (1994) Recent advances in the application of hypnosis to pain management. *Am J Clin Hypnosis*. **37**: 117–27.

59   Price DD (1988) *Psychological and Neural Mechanisms of Pain*. Raven Press, New York.

60   Spanos NP, Burgess CA, Cross PA and MacLeod G (1992) Hypnosis, reporting bias, and suggested negative hallucinations. *J Abnorm Psychol*. **101**: 192–9.

61   Chaves JF and Barber TX (1974) Cognitive strategies, experimenter modeling, and expectation in the attenuation of pain. *J Abnorm Psychol*. **83**: 356–63.

62   O' Grady DJ and Hoffmann C (1984) Hypnosis with children and adolescents in the medical setting. In: W Wester and A Smith (eds) *Clinical Hypnosis: a multidisciplinary approach*. Lippincott, Philadelphia, PA, 181–209.

63   Hilgard J and LeBaron S (1984) *Hypnotherapy of Pain in Children with Cancer*. Kaufman, Los Altos, CA.

64   Levitan A (1990) Setting sun metaphor. In: DC Hammond (ed.) *Handbook of Hypnotic Suggestions and Metaphors*. Norton, New York.

65   Hammond DC (1990) *Handbook of Hypnotic Suggestions and Metaphors*. Norton, New York.

66   Gardner GG (1981) Teaching self-hypnosis to children. *Int J Clin Exp Hypnosis*. **29**: 300–12.

6

Integrated care

Christina Liossi

Introduction

Despite an increasing awareness of the incidence and severity of paediatric acute pain, many children continue to suffer pain and anxiety associated with medical procedures. Traditionally, intervention for medical procedures has focused on either psychological or pharmacological techniques. Few paediatric oncology departments provide their patients with both, and in the paediatric literature there is very little discussion of how to practically implement an integrated, pharmacological/psychological approach.

The purpose of this chapter is to propose and discuss such an integrated treatment approach that can be routinely implemented by healthcare providers when performing medical procedures (painful or not) in the paediatric oncology setting. The chapter begins with a discussion of the advantages and disadvantages of psychological and pharmacological techniques. A summary of the conceptual basis for a multidisciplinary approach and a specific integrated treatment model for the management of pain associated with procedures are then presented. Particular emphasis is placed on the role of psychological factors in the model, and how they can be integrated with pharmacological treatment throughout the phases of a medical procedure. Finally, areas where further research is required are identified.

The pros and cons of psychological and pharmacological interventions

According to Chapman,[1] the basic strategies of symptomatic pain control can be assigned to one of three categories:

1 attenuation or blockade of nociception through intervention at the periphery
2 activation of inhibitory processes that gate nociception at the spinal cord or brainstem
3 interference with the perception, meaning and affect associated with the pain, and/or modification of pain behaviour or pain expression.

Although some therapies for pain may involve all three strategies of pain control, most can be ascribed to one. Non-steroidal anti-inflammatory drugs, physical therapeutic modalities, peripheral neural augmentation techniques and regional analgesia are representatives of the first category of interventions. Pharmacological interventions involving opioids activate nociception, inhibiting neural circuits, and are therefore categorised as the second type of intervention. Psychological interventions are directed at brain processes or the interface between the individual and the environment, and are therefore assigned to the third category.[1] Taking into account the multidimensional nature of pain and the strategies for symptomatic control that are available, the clinician should not expect to find a single pharmacological or psychological treatment for the optimum management of paediatric procedure-related cancer pain, or indeed of any pain. Optimal treatment of pain is always a multimodal process, and no single, narrowly based intervention brings about a comprehensive improvement.

There are certainly both advantages and disadvantages to psychological and pharmacological approaches when administered as separate interventions. Clinicians who are treating pain must assume a realistic stance with regard to the role of psychological interventions. The latter are like medical interventions – they are not effective with every patient. Some patients obtain tremendous pain relief, some clearly find such interventions helpful but are in need of still other methods of relief, some find that they reduce the affective components of pain, making the sensory pain more tolerable, and some patients derive no benefit from them. With regard to the treatment of pain, the clinician who uses psychological interventions should not work in isolation. A multidisciplinary team is ideal, and interdisciplinary co-operation is vitally important. Furthermore, psychological management is of limited applicability to children who are very young (lower age limits range from 3 to 7 years in different centres), severely developmentally delayed, or previously traumatised to a severe degree. Younger children in particular may lack the motivation, cognitive abilities, or both, to use such techniques effectively. Furthermore, if children are referred for psychological interventions when they are already extremely distressed, such interventions can be very difficult or virtually impossible to implement. The availability of expert practitioners is also limited in many centres, and personnel typically need specialised training in order to use techniques such as hypnosis, relaxation training or cognitive therapy.

However, psychological interventions have several attractive features. They are safe, and they do not cause side-effects or drug interactions. Both conscious sedation and general anaesthesia carry a very small but real risk of adverse events. Adult outcome studies suggest that conscious sedation by non-specialists carries a higher risk than general anaesthesia or monitored anaesthetic care (i.e. conscious or deep sedation monitored by anaesthetists).

Psychological intervention techniques can be easily and routinely incorporated into standard medical care, and may make analgesics and sedatives more effective or even unnecessary, further reducing the need for the presence of specialists with sedation or special airway skills. Moreover, parents can be actively involved (if they wish) by assisting their children with the psychological techniques, with all of the benefits that such involvement has for both the child and his or her parents.

In some developing or currency-restricted countries where there are inadequate financial resources, it can be argued that the application of psychological interventions such as those described in this book is a cost-effective and realistic alternative to expensive pharmacological approaches.

Psychological approaches have the additional benefit that they can be generalised to other distressing circumstances. The child who learns coping strategies for the management of invasive procedures may apply their skills to decreasing the distress of other aspects of their treatment, such as managing chemotherapy-related nausea and vomiting.[2] It is suggested that the earlier in the course of the disease a child is exposed to the possibility of psychological coping techniques, the more likely they are to succeed (and more quickly) in using them for desired symptom control.

A very important clinical consideration is the contribution of psychological methods to restoring the patient's sense of self-control, personal efficacy and active participation in their own care. During procedures, the goal of psychological interventions is to shift the child from the relatively passive or helpless state of directly experiencing pain and anxiety, and succumbing to pharmacological and other interventions, to a state of empowerment and control.

Finally, one of the major contributions of psychological treatments (although it is difficult to prove experimentally for both methodological and ethical reasons) when used either alone or as an integral part of pharmacological interventions is their potential to prevent the development and establishment of maladaptive schemata in the children involved, and consequently the development of psychopathology either in childhood or later in life. Children with cancer who receive inadequate psychological support and who are not allowed to take an active part in their treatment, including the management of their pain, are in danger of developing negative thoughts about themselves, their world and their future (the depressive triad) that embody themes of worthlessness, guilt, incompetence, defeat, deprivation, loneliness and hopelessness (*see* Box 6.1).

According to Young,[3] early maladaptive schemata are extremely stable and enduring themes that develop during childhood and are elaborated upon throughout an individual's lifetime. These schemata serve as templates for processing later experience. They provide a basis for screening, coding and evaluating stimuli, orienting oneself psychologically in the world, categorising and interpreting experiences, making predictions, and testing those predictions via behaviour.[4] They develop over the course of numerous experiences, and are adaptive in so far as they facilitate efficient information processing. They enable new information to be linked to old information so that it can be recognised and recalled more readily and appropriate action can be taken as necessary.

Cognitive theories of psychopathology maintain that individuals with emotional disorders have particular schemata that bias them toward perceiving situations in terms of loss, danger or other types of threats to the self. Although such schemata may be relatively dormant at most

---

Box 6.1: The cognitive triad of an adolescent[6.1] with cancer who was receiving inadequate psychological support for medical procedures

- The self is damaged, defective, disabled and impaired (e.g. 'I need others. I cannot function on my own', 'I do not have the resources to cope').
- The world is punishing, blaming, uncaring, unfair, depriving and disappointing (e.g. 'I receive an endless array of procedures and medications').
- The future is painful, fearful, a struggle, more disabling, deteriorating and hopeless (e.g. 'I will spend the rest of my life going in and out of hospital, feeling pain, and being poked and drugged').

6.1   Based on the treatment sessions with an adolescent who had been referred to the therapist for mild depression.

times, they can become activated by the occurrence of certain stressful life events or negative mood states. Once activated, these schemata may dominate an individual's perception of new situations, thus maintaining the emotional state. It therefore makes intuitive sense that by preparing children psychologically for medical procedures and teaching them coping strategies, healthcare professionals can prevent the development of maladaptive, dysfunctional schemata, and consequently prevent the development of psychopathology later in life.

Pharmacological interventions also have advantages. Many effective agents are now available that provide significant amnesia, anxiolysis and analgesia for almost any procedure. When used appropriately, this approach is safe and effective (*see* Chapter 3). A major disadvantage of the pharmacological approach is that anticipatory anxiety is not addressed, thereby increasing the distress that the child experiences (and consequently that of his or her family) while waiting for a procedure. Moreover, amnesia which may result from pharmacological agents has both advantages and disadvantages. Children may not remember that they tolerated the pre-procedure waiting period and the associated anticipatory anxiety and subsequent aspects of the procedure. In essence, they do not remember coping, and this impedes their learning that they are capable of coping with future procedures and generally adverse and stressful situations during the course of their illness and also later in life. This contributes to the development of a sense of self as vulnerable, disabled and impaired, with both short- and long-term consequences in terms of quality of life and psychological distress. Finally, medical and nursing personnel need to be well trained to provide pharmacological interventions safely, because medications used for conscious sedation have potentially adverse effects, such as respiratory depression and loss of protective airway reflexes. Personnel with such appropriate training and experience are not always available.

The integration of pharmacological and psychological techniques maximises the advantages of both approaches, and minimises the disadvantages of either approach when employed alone. Thus the integrated approach combines the best of both interventions to achieve the following goals:

*   to decrease the anticipatory anxiety of the child and his or her family before medical procedures
*   to minimise the child's pain and anxiety and the family's distress during the actual procedure
*   to promote effective coping with subsequent medical procedures and other stressful situations, such as chemotherapy during cancer treatment

- to promote mastery of stressful situations
- to promote an active, adaptive attitude towards life and a view of the self as powerful and competent.

Integrated care in clinical practice

Given that research is providing guidelines for clinicians who care for patients undergoing invasive medical procedures, it is imperative to consider how analgesic interventions (both pharmacological and psychological) can be integrated into mainstream healthcare. The psychological and medical literature is relatively devoid of research that addresses issues related to the implementation of such programmes. In addition, the systematic integration of pharmacological and psychological approaches into actual clinical practice is rare. There are many reasons for this.

Although paediatric oncology centres provide state-of-the-art anti-cancer treatment, psychological care, particularly as an analgesic intervention, is in many cases regarded as being of secondary importance. This lower priority is reflected in the provision of limited resources for psychological support compared with other medical and nursing duties, and in the unsystematic preparation and teaching of staff with regard to the skills necessary for providing psychological care. Difficulties in implementing psychological care in practice reflect the conceptual gap between the predominant philosophy of medicine as aiming to cure disease, and the philosophy of psychology as aiming to care. All health professionals are, at least in theory, keen to stress the significance of psychological support in the holistic care of patients. However, in practice the all-invasive culture of medicine to a great extent determines the resources, activities and managerial structure of hospitals.

Psychological approaches that are used to manage pain and distress during procedures require greater time commitments, separate training sessions, and practice on the part of the child and his or her family – something that is not necessary for pharmacological interventions. The slow process by which psychologists collect information and administer psychological interventions also does not fit well within the busy, fast-paced medical environment. However, psychologists must learn to work faster than might be their normal routine. Patient assessment and treatment sessions need not take hours. Although time constraints are realistic considerations, research has shown that in the care of children with cancer it is important to introduce psychological interventions early and consistently. Children can quickly associate pain and anxiety with their cancer treatment, resulting in poor coping behaviours such as non-compliance. Once developed, these maladaptive behaviours are usually refractory to medical or psychological intervention. The need for all children who are newly diagnosed with cancer to receive training in the use of psychological interventions, and the reality of the availability of various healthcare providers and time constraints, may require a reassessment of delivery of services. Nurses appear to be in a perfect position to provide the majority of psychological care, with other healthcare professionals collaborating and supporting their role in the provision of these services. A standard training programme in psychological coping strategies can be provided by trained nurses, and introduced to all newly diagnosed families. A psychologist could then be available for families who are experiencing complex difficulties in coping.

Lack of systematic interventions for procedural pain can also be understood by looking at the process of change as a stressor to staff, and by studying staff attitudes and perceptions of comprehensive integrated treatment programmes across a variety of dimensions. Indeed, whether it is perceived as positive or negative, change is a stressor. Resistance to changes in practice is real and potentially overwhelming.[5] Introducing new programmes necessitates assessment of the organisational climate and relationships, as well as support from key individuals and groups within any organisation.[6] For changes to be accepted broadly, consistently and expediently, knowledge of scientific data is only one step in the process. Attitudes, beliefs and communication styles all affect the implementation of new practices. However, research indicates[7] that a patient-oriented, integrated pharmacological/psychological intervention for procedural distress can be accepted and used by multidisciplinary staff in a paediatric oncology unit.

McGrath and colleagues[8] suggest that a major reason why pain control therapies, especially the psychological ones, are not routinely used in clinical practice is that many health professionals have not yet shifted their pain paradigm. They continue to utilise the traditional paradigm (i.e. that pain is determined only by the trauma of the procedure, and is relatively benign and brief, that interventions are costly in time and money and that complete pain management is only possible by general anaesthesia). Thomas Kuhn[9] described the scientific paradigm as 'accepted examples of actual scientific practice, examples which include law, theory, application and instrumentation together (that) provide models from which spring particular coherent traditions of scientific research. Men whose research is based on shared paradigms are committed to the same rules and standards for scientific practice'. Furthermore, Barker[10] states that 'A paradigm is a set of rules and regulations (written and unwritten) that does two things: (1) it establishes or defines boundaries; and (2) it tells you how to behave inside the boundaries in order to be successful'. A paradigm never remains static, but rather it changes and evolves as new knowledge is accumulated and ideas are conceived, causing a paradigm shift. The traditional paradigm for managing procedural pain in children should shift to incorporate the new knowledge of what pain is and how it can be assessed and managed adequately.

Medical training seems to produce a less speculative individual than does psychological training.[11] Medical practitioners do not think in terms of theories, paradigm shifts and probabilities, but are more focused towards pragmatic, technical and sometimes impersonal solutions to problems. The potential pitfalls in the relationship between psychological and medical practitioners have received considerable attention, at least in books and reviews aimed at psychologists.[12,13] Differences in training and background, preferences for different research methods and lack of awareness about what other specialties can (and cannot) offer can be so pronounced that effective collaboration is inhibited. These difficulties are only likely to be reduced by more integrated training programmes and joint dissemination of research findings, which are equally accessible to all disciplines.

Integration of input from multiple disciplines has been applied and proved to be highly successful in chronic pain management, and is recommended as the best approach for developing treatment protocols for the optimal management of acute paediatric pain.

Case history 6.1

Helen was a 10-year-old girl with acute myeloid leukaemia. Shorly after the diagnosis she was introduced to the use of hypnosis to help her to undergo procedures with minimal pain and distress during her treatment. She responded well, and she was using hypnosis as the sole anaesthetic for venepunctures, and in combination with pharmacological interventions for lumbar punctures and bone-marrow aspirations. On her own initiative she started to use hypnosis to manage the anticipatory nausea and vomiting and the chemotherapy-related nausea and vomiting that she had to endure during the course of her illness. After the first remission she reported using hypnosis as an ego-strengthening technique, since she had been left behind in school, and also to enhance her performance in her favourite sport (gymnastics). After she relapsed she continued to use hypnosis, and when the anti-cancer treatment was no longer successful she used it during the terminal stage of her illness for managing symptoms such as insomnia and anxiety, and as a way to escape in fantasy from the hospital environment.

How to prepare children with cancer for medical procedures

A comprehensive model for acute pain management needs to incorporate the dynamic interrelationships of physiological, cognitive, emotional, behavioural and contextual factors and the changes between these relationships over time. From this perspective, children in pain, as is true for all individuals, are viewed as active processors of information. They have negative expectations about their own ability and responsibility to exert any control over their pain or distress, and they often view themselves as helpless. Such negative, maladaptive appraisals of their situation and their personal efficacy may reinforce the experience of demoralisation and over-reaction to nociceptive stimulation, and should be addressed by both pharmacological and psychological interventions.

This section will discuss a set of guidelines for the management of paediatric procedure-related cancer pain. The model is consistent and elaborates the guidelines published by the World Health Organisation.[14] The goal is to suggest and describe briefly, based on the existing literature as well as on clinical experience, the specific steps to be taken in the management of pain and distress in young patients who are undergoing medical procedures.

Children must be adequately prepared for all invasive and diagnostic procedures, from finger-pricks to bone-marrow aspirations and imaging scans, and this requires pain and distress prevention to be placed higher up the list of priorities in each child's overall plan of care. Prophylaxis of procedure pain should involve both pharmacological and non-pharmacological approaches (*see* Box 6.2). The specific combination of approaches used should be determined by considering the individual child, the specific procedure, and the needs and preferences of the child and his or her family.

Aggressive pharmacological treatment of a child during their first experience of a painful procedure is necessary in order to prevent the cycle of fear that emerges when that procedure must be performed repeatedly. Psychological approaches should be adopted after the initial diagnostic procedures have been completed.[14]

Box 6.2:   The World Health Organisation (WHO) position[14]

Psychosocial treatment is an integral part of cancer pain treatment. It should be used in all painful or potentially painful situations, often combined with analgesic drug therapy.

Box 6.3: Algorithms for pain management during procedures

1 *Painless procedures, e.g. computerised tomography, magnetic resonance imaging*

   - Individualised preparation
   - When sedation is necessary, chloral hydrate 1 hour before procedure
   - When chloral hydrate is unsuccessful (in an older or developmentally retarded child, or because of an idiosyncratic reaction), and if monitoring facilities are adequate, pentobarbital

2 *Mildly painful procedures, e.g. finger sticks, intravenous cannulation, venepunctures*

   - Individualised preparation
   - Parental presence
   - Grouping of procedures so that repetition – of finger sticks, for example – is not necessary
   - Local anaesthetics:

     – topical anaesthetics
     – buffered lidocaine

   - Behavioural techniques, such as bubble blowing, party blowers, distraction

3 *Moderately painful procedures, e.g. lumbar puncture*

   - Individualised preparation
   - Local anaesthetics:

     – topical anaesthetics
     – buffered lidocaine

   - Behavioural techniques, such as distraction, hypnosis
   - Benzodiazepines (in selected children)

4 *Moderately to severely painful procedures, e.g. bone marrow aspiration, biopsy*

   - Individualised preparation and parental presence
   - Local anaesthetics:

     – topical anaesthetics
     – buffered lidocaine

   - Any drug regimen that produces conscious sedation in a carefully monitored setting. Examples include the following:

     if venous access is established: intravenous midazolam with fentanyl or morphine 5 minutes before the procedure

> *if there is no established venous access*: oral midazolam with morphine *or* oral diazepam with intramuscular ketamine *or* general anaesthesia
>
> Reprinted with permission from WHO (1998) *Cancer Pain Relief and Palliative Care in Children.* WHO, Geneva, pp. 57–8.

Phases of the medical procedure

Every medical procedure, painful or not, essentially consists of four phases:

- anticipatory phase
- preparatory phase
- procedural phase
- recovery phase.

These are described in turn below. Before these phases, health professionals have generally become familiar with the child and his or her family, they know the child's medical history, they have thoroughly assessed the psychological state of the child and his or her family, and they have jointly designed with them an individualised analgesic protocol for the child. The child will already have been taught psychological interventions for pain management.

Anticipatory phase

The anticipatory phase involves assessing and preparing the child and their parents for the procedure. During this phase, vital information is obtained for the implementation of both pharmacological and psychological interventions. For the pharmacological intervention, this consists primarily of a brief physical examination and familiarisation with the child's medical history. For the psychological intervention, the same or a different professional should find out the child's knowledge and expectations about the procedure, and if the child has any misconceptions these should be corrected. In addition, it is helpful to inquire into the child's previous experiences of medical procedures. Finally, the anxiety level of both the parent and the child should be evaluated, and the ability of both to cope with the procedure should be assessed. This information will assist the healthcare provider in determining whether the parent will be able to help the child by coaching him or her in the utilisation of psychological techniques, or whether medical or nursing personnel will have to provide most of the psychological support.

Healthcare professionals should, if possible, meet and evaluate the child and his or her parent in a room other than the treatment room. Obtaining information from the child and their parent in a less intimidating atmosphere, and also performing the physical examination away from the treatment room, helps to decrease anxiety.

The initiation of the practice of appropriate psychological interventions during this phase (before the child enters the treatment room) decreases anticipatory anxiety. In addition, it is preferable to engage the child in psychological techniques before they enter the treatment room, because their aroused emotional state may impede their ability to attend to this material after entering the room. As a general rule, the utilisation of psychological interventions at the outset is much more effective (pre-empting distress) than attempting to intervene after the child has become terrified.

Preparatory phase

After the evaluation, the child is taken to the procedure room. This signifies the transition to the preparatory phase, which is the period just before the actual procedure, when final preparations are necessary (e.g. the child undressing, placement of monitors). It is of critical importance to focus attention immediately on both the child and the parent upon entry to the treatment room, and to do everything possible to reduce distress associated with entry into this new and potentially stressful environment. Being well organised (e.g. having all consent forms signed and all medications drawn up, making sure that all equipment for the procedure is ready, and keeping potentially frightening equipment such as needles out of view) ensures that attention is directed towards the child and the parent when they enter the room. Continuing psychological interventions on entering the treatment room helps to prevent or reduce the child's anxiety (e.g. blowing bubbles, introducing new books, facilitating the use of hypnosis or cognitive interventions) and create a supportive atmosphere. One person, such as the physician who will be performing the procedure, can take the role of the co-ordinator by instructing the child, the parent and other members of the team on appropriate action. This contributes both to the efficiency of the procedure and to the maintenance of a calm, relaxed, child-friendly atmosphere. Parents should be included in this if they wish, and encouraged to coach their child in the use of coping strategies.

The preparation phase often includes 'supporting' procedures – that is, procedures that are necessary for the main procedure. For example, for a bone-marrow aspiration, an intravenous insertion prior to sedation can be painful, and is often the most distressing aspect of the entire procedure.

Reducing anxiety associated with these supporting procedures by using psychological techniques, rather than pharmacological means, decreases the overall amount of medication given and thus decreases recovery time. Techniques of pain control should be applied in advance of the painful stimulus whenever possible. This pre-emptive approach helps to minimise the emotional problems of fear and anxiety, prevents the 'wind-up' phenomenon of central nervous system sensitisation to noxious stimuli and tissue release of pain mediators, ameliorates the stress response and reduces the subsequent anaesthetic and analgesic requirements.[15] A multimodal approach to pain prevention which includes psychological methods should be the basis of acute pain prevention.

Procedural phase

The procedural phase is the phase in which the main procedure is performed. Pharmacological agents are utilised for this phase of most invasive procedures, but it may be possible to use psychological intervention alone for less invasive or non-invasive procedures, or most often a combination of pharmacological and psychological approaches. The latter combination has been tested successfully with adult patients undergoing percutaneous, vascular and renal procedures[16] and plastic surgery,[17] and has resulted in significant reductions in the medication required for conscious sedation and a decreased incidence of adverse effects. Lang and colleagues[16] randomised 241 patients undergoing percutaneous vascular and renal procedures to receive intra-operative standard care, structured attention or self-hypnotic relaxation. All of the patients had access to patient-controlled intravenous analgesia with fentanyl and midazolam. Pain increased linearly with procedure time in the standard group (gradient of 0.09 in pain score/15 minutes, $P < 0.0001$) and the attention group (gradient 0.04/15 minutes, $P = 0.0425$), but the graph remained flat in the hypnosis group. Anxiety decreased over time in all three groups, with gradients of -0.04 (standard), -0.07 (attention) and -0.11 (hypnosis). Drug use in the standard group (1.9 units) was significantly higher than that in the attention and hypnosis groups (0.8 and 0.9 units, respectively). One hypnosis patient became haemodynamically unstable, compared with 10 patients ($P = 0.0041$) in the attention group and 12 patients ($P = 0.0009$) in the standard group. Procedure times were significantly shorter in the hypnosis group (61 minutes) than in the standard group (78 minutes, $P = 0.0016$), with an intermediate value for procedure duration in the attention group (67 minutes).

Psychological interventions are also aimed at reducing parental anxiety associated with sedation and anaesthesia. Many parents are more anxious about the anaesthesia or sedation than they are about the medical procedure. If the parents are present during induction of sedation, it is essential to provide them with information about the procedure and to prepare them for 'normal' physiological responses that may occur, and to support them. For example, the dissociation associated with ketamine or the rapidity of onset of propofol (sometimes accompanied by a short period of agitation) can be quite distressing to parents. In addition, non-verbal communication (a warm pat on the shoulder) and verbal communication ('we will take good care of Mary, she will be fine') should be used to comfort the parents as they leave their child.

Healthcare professionals should be aware that pharmacological interventions sometimes have nothing more than a placebo effect, and therefore they could easily be replaced by cheaper psychological interventions. Abbott and Fowler-Kerry[18] assessed in a double-blind placebo-controlled study the efficacy of a refrigerant topical anaesthetic (Fluro-ethyl) in reducing injection pain in preschool children receiving routine diphtheria–pertussis–tetanus (DPT) immunisations. They found that both the refrigerant spray and the placebo spray significantly reduced injection pain, and in fact were equally effective in reducing such pain. The investigators concluded that utilising positive suggestion statements (e.g. 'This may really help the needle hurt less') often enhances the pain-relieving effects of pharmacological pain interventions, and the two approaches should be used together.

Recovery phase

The recovery phase is the time period after the completion of the procedure. The child should be monitored in the appropriate environment, with adequate nursing coverage to handle potential problems. In addition to physiological recovery, the child's emotional recovery from a procedure is crucial. Thus psychological interventions should continue to be utilised after the procedure is over. Providing an opportunity to recover from the stressful experience helps the child to feel a sense of mastery over the situation and to remember coping, and it prevents the development of negative expectations about future procedures.

Case history 6.2

Steven was a 7-year-old boy who was receiving general anaesthetic for his bone-marrow aspirations. He was extremely distressed during the pre-procedure intravenous placement, and was always sedated as quickly as possible. In most cases he was awakening distressed and was trying to pull out the intravenous attachment. This caused some surprise among the medical and nursing personnel involved in his care, but very soon they realised that Steven's reaction was not unexpected, because his last memory before being sedated would be that of being restrained for the intravenous placement and being anxious. As soon as they realised this, one of the nurses started to use psychological interventions (i.e. distraction) with Steven before and during the intravenous insertion and during the recovery from the general anaesthetic phase, and this resulted in him being able to undergo procedures calmly.

Case history 6.3

Graham was a 9-year-old boy with non-Hodgkin's lymphoma. The analgesic protocols that were used throughout his cancer treatment for the management of venepuncture, lumbar puncture and bone-marrow aspiration are shown in Boxes 6.4 and 6.5

Box 6.4: Analgesic protocol for venepunctures and lumbar punctures

Aims/goals

- To minimise pain and distress during venepunctures and lumbar punctures
- To facilitate mastery of the procedure and increased self-efficacy

Phases

Anticipatory
60 minutes before the procedure: application of Eutectic Mixture of Local Anaesthetics (EMLA) to the site of the procedure, brief assessment of the psychological status of the patient and his parent, and provision of information
A few minutes before the procedure: initiation of the use of psychological techniques (e.g. hypnosis or bubble blowing)
Preparatory: continue using psychological techniques
Procedural: continue using psychological techniques, with the parent acting as a coach
Recovery: continue using psychological techniques; the family is praised for the success of the procedure and their active participation

Anticipatory phase

- Establish rapport with the family
- Assess the current physical and psychological status of the patient and the psychological status of the parent who will accompany the child to the treatment room
- Determine the type and level of pharmacological and psychological intervention that is required and desired, depending on the specific procedure and the individual child and his or her family
- Share your pain management protocol with the child and his or her family
- Encourage the child to start practising his or her coping skills

Preparatory phase

- Be organised
- Reduce the distress of the child and their family on entry to the treatment room
- Encourage the child to continue practising their coping strategies
- Encourage the parents to 'coach' their children if they wish to do so
- Perform 'supporting' procedures if necessary

Procedural phase

- Minimise pain and anxiety by the most effective combination of pharmacological and psychological techniques following the protocol that you have devised for the individual child
- Ensure the patient's safety by means of the necessary monitoring equipment and the presence of appropriately trained personnel
- Make a positive psychological impact on both the child and their parents, and ensure that healthcare professionals are involved in the care of the patient and his or her family and do not perform their tasks 'mechanically'

Recovery phase

- Monitor the child in the appropriate environment and with the appropriate professionals present
- Encourage the child to continue to use his or her coping skills
- Answer any questions/correct any misconceptions of the child and parent if necessary
- Praise the child and his or her parents for the fact that their coping efforts have contributed to a successful procedure

Figure 6.1:   The integrated approach to the management of paediatric procedure-related cancer pain.

Box 6.5:   Analgesic protocol for bone-marrow aspirations and trephines

Aims/goals

- To minimise pain and distress during bone-marrow aspirations and trephines
- To facilitate mastery of the procedure and increased self-efficacy

Phases

Anticipatory
12 hours before the procedure: physical and psychological assessment of the child and his parent; provision of information about the requirements of general anaesthetic
A few minutes before the procedure: initiation of the use of psychological techniques (i.e. hypnosis)
Preparatory: administration of 'supporting' procedures; continue using psychological techniques
Procedural: general anaesthesia
Recovery: monitoring of the patient; resume use of psychological techniques; the family is praised for the success of the procedure and their active participation

---

The role of the healthcare professionals

When performing painful procedures, depersonalisation is one defence mechanism used by staff as a way of distancing themselves from the patient's and family's distress. With a larger repertoire of pharmacological and psychological resources for procedural pain, staff may experience fewer feelings of depersonalisation. Moreover, the presence of a team-oriented, accepted programme for procedural pain helps staff to remain actively connected to patients, and may enhance their ability to function empathically while performing unpleasant but necessary invasive procedures.[6]

The physician is an important potential influence on the child's distress, but has been relatively neglected in the literature. Effective physician–patient communication during office visits has been found to be related to a variety of important patient outcomes, including patient satisfaction, knowledge about illness, anxiety, and compliance with medical recommendations.[19] However, most of these findings are based on observations of physician interactions with adult patients or, in paediatric studies, on physician–parent interactions.[20] There has been surprisingly little study of physician–child communication in general or physician–child interactions specifically during medical procedures.[19,21] The few studies that have examined physician or nurse behaviours during invasive medical procedures have looked at parent, nurse and physician behaviours in combination,[22,23] rather than directly comparing physician and/or nurse and parent behaviour.

In studies of interactions between adult patients and physicians, patient satisfaction has been shown to be related to 'socio-emotional' physician verbalisations which communicate understanding and acceptance.[24] 'Task-oriented' physician variables, such as information giving, asking questions and technical competence, have also been found to be related to adult patient satisfaction. Furthermore, task-oriented and socio-emotional variables appear to be closely interrelated, in that task-oriented variables are also viewed by patients as reflecting caring on the part of the physician.[25,26] Based on this model, for adult patients to feel satisfied with their interaction with a physician, some minimal amount of both task-oriented and socio-emotional interchange must take place. Although this has not been studied with regard to children, it is reasonable to assume that task-oriented and socio-emotional variables would also be important to children's subjective experience of a medical procedure. Thus for a child to perceive the physician as understanding and accepting, and to experience any task-oriented physician behaviours, the physician must interact with the child.

Subsequent research could consider the relative importance of socio-emotional vs. task-oriented interactions, as well as the timing and appropriateness of physician behaviours. In future research it would also be important to determine whether more physician–child interaction is always better, or whether there is simply a minimal amount of interaction necessary to establish a satisfactory physician–child interaction and facilitate the child's attempts to use coping strategies. One approach would be to manipulate the physician–child interaction experimentally in order to explore whether the amount and type of that child interaction affects children's distress during the medical procedure and influences their efforts to control the distress caused by the procedure by means of psychological techniques.

Future studies should also consider whether the unique qualities of physicians and nurses make them more effective agents of change than parents in the context of invasive medical procedures. There appears to be considerable potential for physicians and nurses to become more effective in this situation in terms of the overall amount of interaction, as well as possible improvements in the timing and/or appropriateness of interactions with the child.

Parents' role in pain treatment

A particularly important area of preparation of children for invasive procedures is the involvement of primary caregivers (normally parents or close relatives). There is some debate as to whether parents should be present when their children are undergoing procedures. There is little doubt that children may be more disruptive if their parents are present.[27,28] Observations of parent–child interactions during medical procedures suggest that parents may influence child distress by modelling distress behaviour and/or that parents may differentially reinforce distress behaviours. For example, children's distress has been observed to be greater when their parents engage in behaviours that appear to communicate anxiety, such as agitation[29,30] and apology.[23] Child distress has also been shown to be positively associated with parental behaviours that are responses to child distress behaviours, such as parental reassurance,[22,23,30,31] explanation,[31–33] giving control to the child (e.g. 'Tell me when you are ready'), and criticism.[23] Healthcare professionals should discourage parents from engaging in these behaviours which have been found to be most closely associated with child distress.

Almost all children want their parents to be present during painful procedures.[34] Likewise, almost all parents would prefer to be present when their children are undergoing a painful procedure. Most parents report that they are active in providing comfort and information to their children before and during procedures.[35] However, parents are not usually prepared for painful procedures. When parents are trained, they can be of considerable assistance to their children. Parental use of distraction appears to be associated with lower levels of child distress during general paediatric examinations,[29,30] venepunctures[33] and bone-marrow aspiration and lumbar puncture procedures.[23,31]

Parents should be trained, if they wish, in psychological interventions to assist their children. When trained together with their children, they can play a supportive role before, after and in some cases during medical procedures. This role would serve to decrease the sense of helplessness that is often expressed by parents, by allowing them to participate in activities which could serve to reduce their child's distress. Furthermore, parents can also introduce psychological techniques at home, to help to facilitate ongoing communication between parent and child. Parental demonstration of effective coping and stress management at home can provide the child with support and reassurance. In this respect, parental intervention may be a useful adjunct to child treatment.[36] Overall, for parents to play a full role in helping children with pain, changes must be made in professional attitudes, educational material and organisation of services. Research on different aspects of parents' role in pain assessment and management is also needed. The importance of the family in ensuring the general health and well-being of children was recognised in the World Declaration on the Survival, Protection and Development of Children at the World Summit for Children:

> The family has the primary responsibility for the nurturing and protection of children from infancy to adolescence ... and all institutions of society and other caregivers to nurture and care for children in a family environment.[37]

How can the integrated approach be implemented in clinical practice?

Education

Professionals

Studies have shown that one of the main reasons for poor paediatric pain management is a lack of education of staff, parents and children. Myths and misconceptions persist. Medical and nursing students have often received very little formal training in paediatric pain management, but are expected to prescribe and administer analgesia to children. As a result, staff often express undue concern about side-effects, and tend to use inadequate doses of analgesic drugs. Their knowledge of psychological intervention techniques is usually even more limited.

Practice can be changed by education. This is illustrated by the changes in perception and practice among paediatric anaesthetists who were surveyed in 1988, and again in 1995. In 1988, only 27% of the respondents were using a local anaesthetic for minor surgery, whereas in 1995 the overwhelming majority (99%) did so.[38] Studies also show that nurses who have received training in the management of pain in children identify more indicators of pain,[39] use more pain management strategies[40] and give more narcotics than those who have not received such training.

Educational efforts can be incorporated at various points and in varying formats throughout the health professional's career, in the undergraduate curriculum and in continuing formal postgraduate education. In addition, information can be introduced via review articles in journals and textbooks, and through practice guidelines. The International Association for the Study of Pain (IASP) has developed pain-related curricula for incorporation into the overall undergraduate curricula of medical, dental, nursing and pharmacy schools. In addition, occupational therapist/physical therapist curricula and a psychology curriculum are available. Unfortunately, given the vast amount of material to be taught and the limited time available, it is unclear whether the IASP curriculum has been fully incorporated into the overall undergraduate curriculum of any academic institution.

Clinical practice guidelines have been and should continue to be developed by a number of professional societies and governmental and regulatory agencies, to address the widespread belief that clinicians require more detailed and usable information than traditional lectures allow. Such guidelines theoretically present an information package, developed by experts, that weights and codifies the literature and makes it clinically relevant. Guidelines allow clinicians to carry in their pockets a step-by-step approach to a clinical problem, which is endorsed by national authorities. Surveys of the implementation and efficacy of previously developed guidelines (not necessarily those developed for pain) have been disheartening, as it appears that guidelines do not often change practice patterns. A number of explanations have been posited. Clinicians have suggested that some guidelines are too scientific and not applicable to typical clinical settings, or that they are too abstract, and as a result are not user-friendly. Others have suggested that the problem is less to do with the content of the guidelines than with the fact that they have been developed by national and international experts who are not known by the clinicians and who, as a result, are less likely to be believed than local experts on whom clinicians have traditionally depended for information, whom they trust, and whom they assume are familiar with local standards.

Patients and their families

The education of patients and their families can foster a desire for change and put pressure on healthcare providers. Such pressure, especially in a managed care environment, can potentially alter practice patterns.

Regulatory interventions

Although educational efforts allow for change in knowledge and attitudes, stronger measures to precipitate change are often necessary.

Regulatory activities to mandate change and monitor practice have had an important role, and continue to do so. Such activities can be undertaken at a local institutional, national or international level. Clearly, administrative and regulatory efforts can affect the adequacy of pain management.

The multidisciplinary team

The multidisciplinary team is one of the cornerstones for the implementation of the integrated approach. In the multidisciplinary case conference, each professional involved in the care of a particular child presents his or her findings and recommendations, typically in a round-table discussion. As the professionals report their findings, a conceptualisation of the particular case evolves. All members play an equally instrumental role in the case conceptualisation. By completion of the round-table review, a tentative decision is reached and presented to the group for consensus review.

Although the multidisciplinary approach has a scientific basis in both epistemological and clinical outcome research, much has still to be learned about its dynamics and the best ways in which to use it in clinical settings. Many practical challenges also accompany the implementation of such an approach, and at times these make its effective management complex and difficult.

The strategy of flexible roles also presents difficulties. For such an approach to work, it is essential that the various team members recognise the limitations of their knowledge and skills, and do not simply apply what appears to be a 'common-sense' approach to problems. This requires a highly skilled group that works with the best available empirical knowledge and clearly defined treatment goals. A basic understanding of the principles and techniques of each discipline, as well as respect for the contribution of each team member, is critical. A prerequisite for successful team collaboration in the management of pain is the recognition that each team member has something different to contribute, and that no one approach is necessarily better than another.

Box 6.6:   The characteristics of effective multidisciplinary teams
- Functioning under a shared model of the task and team
- Continuous monitoring of performance against well-defined objectives
- Mechanisms in place for self-correction of errors and conflict resolution
- Flexibility and willingness to reconsider the model of care in the light of new evidence

Working as a multidisciplinary team is crucial for the successful implementation of an integrated programme, and it must be an ongoing process, with all team members continually striving to develop and improve their skills.

Research considerations

Suggestions for future research have already been mentioned throughout this book. This section discusses some new lines of research that could be followed, and summarises the most important and clinically useful research questions in the area of procedure-related cancer pain, with an emphasis on psychological research.

Research has demonstrated that a number of psychological interventions have been effective in alleviating the distress that children experience while undergoing painful medical procedures. Most interventions are presented to all children in a similar manner with the assumption that they will benefit equally from a particular intervention programme. In addition, research in this area has tended to evaluate whether one intervention is superior to another in reducing or preventing distress-related behaviour in children. Future research needs to move beyond merely demonstrating the efficacy of a given intervention, to attempting to identify criteria for matching interventions to specific patient characteristics (e.g. cognitive development, coping predisposition) in order to determine which children respond more favourably to a particular treatment strategy. Ideally, children could be matched to the most appropriate intervention for them based on factors such as age, coping style or personal preference.

The effective components of the interventions also need to be identified. It is clear that the research focus should become sharper. A related issue for future research is an examination of the mechanisms (biological as well as psychological) underlying interventions that have been found to be effective, such as hypnosis. Rather than conducting ever larger replication studies, a more appropriate strategy might be to conduct carefully designed analyses of specific biological changes associated with particular psychological treatments. In this way it is possible to conduct research that is theoretically driven and clinically relevant without burdening the patient or disrupting ongoing medical treatment.

Another area that requires further research is an investigation of the timing of interventions (proximity to the aversive medical event) and the timing of the assessment period (before, during or after the event) and their differential impact on the child's behaviour. Moreover, advances in paediatric pain assessment and management have increasingly been achieved in recent years, but there is still much work to be done, especially with regard to establishing the psychometric properties of existing instruments.

Box 6.7 outlines a set of major issues that future research in the area of procedure-related pain must address. At the very least, future studies must have greater methodological rigour, including a clear definition of the target population and the content of the procedure, and a clear description of the interventions used, together with the circumstances, timing and duration of their use, and well-defined outcome measures.

Box 6.7:   Issues for future research in paediatric procedure-related cancer pain

- Pain assessment (development of instruments)
- Pain measurement tools (development of new tools and establishment of the psychometric properties of the existing ones)
- Pain and education (current status, necessary modifications)
- Multidisciplinary approaches to pain management
- Pharmacological intervention modalities
- Psychological interventions (randomised controlled trials)

Greater methodological rigour in:

> details of content, timing and duration of interventions
> selection and definition of outcome variables pertinent to specific types of procedures
> clarity in theoretical linkage between strategies employed and anticipated outcomes
> measurement of both sensory and affective dimensions of pain

Comparative studies:

> psychological vs. pharmacological vs. integrated
> audiotaped vs. *in vivo*
> standardised vs. individually tailored
> brief vs. extended

- Evaluation of optimal matching between the type of procedure, type of patient and type of specific integrated treatment strategy
- A broader range of variables potentially modifying individual differences, including hypnotic ability, cognitive level, coping style, coping demands and previous medical experiences

---

In addition, individual difference factors must be carefully assessed when evaluating outcome, and at the very minimum a description must be provided of the types of coping skills that are required for the procedure for which the patient is being prepared. Finally, research is needed to compare the efficacy of various strategies. This should be undertaken across multiple institutions to ensure that an adequate number of individuals are studied, and to control for variations in setting and therapeutic style, thus ensuring that the findings are generalisable.

There are many strategies available to the researcher who wishes to contribute to our knowledge of pain. One of the least used methods in our field has been multicentre studies. The major advantage of multicentre trials is the accumulation of large number of patients for study. Numerous commentators have noted the dangers of generalising from trials of inadequate sample size. However, multicentre trials present serious challenges with regard to obtaining co-operation and maintaining protocol fidelity. Most paediatric cancer is treated according to protocols designed by collaborative groups. It is widely agreed that the major advances that have been made in the treatment of paediatric cancer have been due in part to the many careful collaborative trials completed by these groups. A similar approach to pain research is very likely to be equally beneficial for patients and their families.

Conclusion

> Despite enormous advances in knowledge of cancer pain relief in children, serious challenges remain in clinical practice. There is a wide gap between what is known and what is practised. Healthcare workers lack up-to-date information about pain systems, methods of pain assessment, and effective means of relieving cancer pain. The highest priority now and in the immediate future must be the application of existing knowledge on relief of children's cancer pain to clinical practice.[14]

It is clear that children's pain has historically been undertreated, and that there is now a plethora of information on how to treat pain in children. It would seem intuitively obvious, therefore, that to improve pain management one would merely need to present this information in appropriate medical forums to practitioners and they could then immediately incorporate it into their patient care. However, it appears that few programmes have been developed, implemented and evaluated in terms of their ability to provide a proactive integrated service to children and their families.

Eliciting behavioural change in medical practice is always complex, and the area of pain management presents a unique challenge. The new information on pain management requires a shift in the conceptual framework of pain, and not merely new ways of treating pain. Bridging the gap between research studies and the daily practice of hospital staff is vital, and the challenge for paediatric healthcare providers in the twenty-first century is not only to be informed about the current literature on pain control, but also most importantly to implement theory and research findings in day-to-day patient management.[14]

Pharmacotherapy is an important treatment approach for acute pain, but it is best utilised in a multidisciplinary setting together with psychological interventions aimed at decreasing suffering and increasing functional and personal autonomy. To assume that medication alone will resolve the complex psychosocial stressors with which the child with cancer is attempting to cope is both naive and simplistic. Thus there is no single way to treat procedure-related pain, and the most successful therapies integrate the best efforts of many disciplines.

It is critical in the course of a child's illness that the child, their family and healthcare professionals know that the child is being helped to be as comfortable as possible, and that his or her emotional and physical well-being are addressed by utilising all of the available empirically supported interventions. Long after memories of the battle against cancer have faded, anguish and guilt may be considerable if the child is remembered as having lived their life in distress, or if they continue as a survivor to suffer the psychological consequences of inadequate pain management.

References

1   Chapman CR (1984) New directions in the understanding and management of pain. *Soc Sci Med.* **19**: 1261–77.

2   Hawkins PJ, Liossi C, Ewart BW, Hatira P, Kosmidis VH and Varvutsi M (1995) Hypnotherapy for control of anticipatory nausea and vomiting in children with cancer: preliminary findings. *Psycho-Oncology.* **4**: 101–6.

3   Young JE (1994) *Cognitive Therapy for Personality Disorders: a schema-focused approach.* Professional Resource Press, Sarasota, FL.

4   Beck AT (1976) *Cognitive Therapy and the Emotional Disorders.* International Universities Press, New York.

5   Kazak AE, Blackall G, Himelstein B, Brophy P and Daller R (1995) Producing systemic change in pediatric practice: an intervention protocol for reducing stress during painful procedures. *Fam Syst Med.* **13**: 173–85.

6 Kazak AE, Blackall GF, Boyer BA *et al.* (1996) Implementing a pediatric leukemia intervention for procedural pain: the impact on staff. *Fam Syst Health.* **14**: 43–56.

7 Liossi C and Hatira P (unpublished data) Pharmacological versus a combination of psychological and pharmacological interventions in the alleviation of procedure-related pain in paediatric oncology patients.

8 McGrath PA, Cohen DE, Fowler-Kerry S and McIntosh N (1996) Controlling children's pain: a practical approach to assessment and management. In: JN Campbell (ed.) *Pain 1996: an updated review. Refresher Course Syllabus.* IASP Press, Seattle.

9 Kuhn TS (1970) *The Structure of Scientific Revolutions* (2e). University of Chicago Press, Chicago.

10 Barker JA (1992) *Paradigms: the business of discovering the future.* Harper Collins Publishers Inc., New York.

11 Kingsbury SJ (1987) Cognitive differences between clinical psychologists and psychiatrists. *Am Psychol.* **42**: 152–6.

12 Drotar D (1989) Psychological research in paediatric settings: lessons from the field. *J Pediatr Psychol.* **14**: 63–74.

13 Tweney RD and Budzynski CA (2000) The scientific status of American psychology in 1900. *Am Psychol.* **55**: 1014–17.

14 World Health Organisation (1998) *Cancer Pain Relief and Palliative Care in Children.* World Heath Organisation, Geneva.

15 Morton NS (1998) *Acute Paediatric Pain Management. A practical guide.* WB Saunders, Philadelphia, PA.

16 Lang EV, Benotsch EG, Fick LJ *et al.* (2000) Adjunctive non-pharmacological analgesia for invasive medical procedures: a randomised trial. *Lancet.* **355**: 1486–90.

17 Faymonville ME, Fisstte J, Mambourg PH, Roediger L, Joris J and Lamy M (1995) Hypnosis as adjunct therapy in conscious sedation for plastic surgery. *Region Anesth.* **20**: 145–51.

18 Abbott K and Fowler-Kerry S (1995) The use of a topical refrigerant anaesthetic to reduce injection pain in children. *J Pain Symp Manage.* **10**: 584–90.

19 Pantell RH and Lewis CC (1986) Physician communication with paediatric patients: a theoretical and empirical analysis. *Adv Dev Behav Pediatrics.* **7**: 65–119.

20 Finney JW, Brophy CJ, Friman PC *et al.* (1990) Promoting parent–provider interaction during young children's health supervision visits. *J Appl Behav Anal.* **23**: 207–13.

21 Rifkin L, Wolf MH, Lewis CC and Pantell RH (1988) Children's perceptions of physicians and medical care: two measures. *J Pediatr Psychol.* **13**: 247–54.

22 Blount RL, Corbin SM, Sturges JW, Wolfe VV, Prater JM and James LD (1989) The relationship between adults' behavior and child coping and distress during BMA/LP procedures: a sequential analysis. *Behav Ther.* **20**: 585–601.

23 Blount RL, Sturges JW and Powers SW (1990) Analysis of child and adult behavioral variations by phase of medical procedure. *Behav Ther.* **21**: 33–48.

24 Stewart M and Roter D (eds) (1989) *Communicating with Medical Patients.* Sage, Newbury Park, CA.

25 Galassi JP, Schanberg R and Ware WB (1992) The Patient Reactions Assessment: a brief measure of the quality of the patient–provider medical relationship. *Psychol Assess.* **4**: 346–51.

26 Roter D (1989) Which facets of communication have strong effects on outcome? A meta-analysis. In: M Stewart and D Roter (eds) *Communicating with Medical Patients.* Sage, Newbury Park, CA.

27 Gonzalez JC, Routh DK, Saab PG and Armstrong FD (1989) Effects of parent presence on children's reactions to injections: behavioral, physiological and subjective aspects. Special issue: pediatric pain, distress and intervention. *J Pediatr Psychol.* **14**: 449–62.

28 Shaw EG and Routh DK (1982) Effect of mother presence on children's reaction to aversive procedures. *J Pediatr Psychol.* **7**: 33–42.

29 Bush JP and Cockrell CS (1987) Maternal factors predicting behaviors in the pediatric clinic. *J Pediatr Psychol.* **12**: 505–18.

30 Bush JP, Melamed BG and Sheras PL *et al.* (1986) Mother–child patterns of coping with anticipatory medical stress. *Health Psychol.* **5**: 137–57.

31 Dahlquist LM, Power TG, Cox CN and Fernbach DJ (1994) Parenting and child distress during cancer procedures: a multidimensional assessment. *Children's Health Care.* **23**: 149–66.

32 Jacobsen P, Manne S, Gorfinkle K, Schorr O, Rapkin B and Redd W (1990) Analysis of child and parent activity during painful medical procedures. *Health Psychol.* **9**: 559–76.

33 Manne SL, Jacobsen PB and Redd WH (1992) Assessment of acute pediatric pain: do child self-report, parent ratings and nurse ratings measure the same phenomenon? *Pain.* **48**: 45–52.

34 Ross DM and Ross SA (1988) *Childhood Pain: current issues, research and management.* Urban and Schwarzenberg, Baltimore, MD.

35 Caty S, Ellerton ML and Ritchie JA (1984) Coping in hospitalized children: analysis of published case studies. *Nurs Res.* **33**: 277–82.

36 LaMontagne L, Wells N, Hepworth J, Johnson B and Manes R (1999) Parent coping and child distress behaviors during invasive procedures for childhood cancer. *J Pediatr Oncol Nurs.* **16**: 3–12.

37 United Nations Children's Fund (UNICEF) (1991) *The State of the World's Children.* Oxford University Press, Oxford.

38 De Lima J, Lloyd-Thomas AR, Howard RF, Sumner E and Quinn TM (1996) Infant and neonatal pain: anaesthetists' perceptions and prescribing patterns. *BMJ.* **313**: 787.

39 Coffman S, Alvarez Y, Pyngolil M, Petit R, Hall C and Smyth M (1997) Nursing assessment and management of pain in critically ill children. *Heart Lung.* **26**: 221–8.

40 McCain GC and Morwessel NJ (1995) Pediatric nurses' knowledge and practice related to infant pain. *Issues Compr Pediatr Nurs.* **18**: 277–86.

Index